D0918450

Try to Remember

Try to Remember

Psychiatry's Clash over
Meaning, Memory, and Mind

by

Paul R. McHugh, M.D.

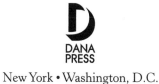

DANA
PRESS

New York • Washington, D.C.

DANA
PRESS

The Dana Foundation
745 Fifth Avenue, Suite 900
New York, NY 10151

900 15th Street NW
Washington, D.C. 20005

DANA is a federally registered trademark.

ISBN-13: 978-1-932594-39-3

This publication is designed to provide accurate and authoritative information in regard to the
subject matter covered. It is sold with the understanding that the publisher is not engaged in
rendering professional services. If professional advice or other expert assistance is required, the
services of a competent professional person should be sought.

Library of Congress Cataloging-in-Publication Data
    McHugh, Paul R. (Paul Rodney), 1931-
        Try to remember : psychiatry's clash over meaning, memory, and mind / by Paul R.
    McHugh.
            p. ; cm.
        Includes bibliographical references.
        ISBN 978-1-932594-39-3 (cloth : alk. paper)
        1. False memory syndrome. 2. Recovered memory. 3. Psychiatric errors. I. Title.
        [DNLM: 1. Repression. 2. Psychiatry—history. 3. Psychotherapy—methods. WM
        193.5.R4 M151t 2008]
    RC455.2.F35M35 2008
    616.89'14—dc22
                        2008036331

Text design by William Stilwell
Cover design by Moiré Studio

www.dana.org

In memory of Martin Orne—
thoughtful scientist, gracious teacher,
supportive colleague, devoted clinician

Life is short,
The art long,
The occasion instant,
Experiment perilous,
Decision difficult.

—Hippocrates of Cos

(an epigraph on Building D facing the quadrangle of Harvard Medical School)

Contents

Acknowledgments

Clinicians always need help. Their views must be transformed by the sciences that surround their art and their practices evaluated by results. This is hardly a new idea—see the epigraph of Hippocrates beneath which I walked all unnoticing during my most formative years.

Several people who worked directly with me in the adventures described herein have been identified with gratitude in the text, but many others also helped me write this book. They include Chris Barden, Fred Berlin, Jason Brandt, Maggie Bruck, Terry Campbell, Michael Clark, Frederick Crews, Midge Decter, Raymond DePaulo, David Edwin, Joseph Epstein, Janet Fetkewicz, Peter Freyd, Morton Goldberg, Angela Guarda, Rudolf Hoehn-Saric, Amy Huberman, Jim Hudson, Mark Lasswell, Robert Leavitt, SS, Harold Lief, Beth Loftus, Francis McMahon, Richard McNally, Harold Merskey, Frank Mondimore, Timothy Moran, Richard Ofshe, Emily Orne, Martin Orne, Michael Packenham, August Piper, Norman Podhoretz, Harrison Pope, Alan Romanoski, Gerald Rosen, Patricia Santora, James Shea, Margaret Singer, Phillip Slavney, Glenn Treisman, Simon Wessely, and Tom Wolfe. In one way or another, each provided me with important thoughts, concepts, and corrections derived from their own experience and knowledge with psychiatry, with our culture, and with writing. Of course, all errors that abide despite their efforts to help remain my responsibility.

Four people were essential to the enterprise. Pam Freyd first suggested the project and then most patiently supported it. Clare McHugh, in what was a delightful yearlong collaboration, helped me put down an accessible draft, smoothing away as much of my professional jargon as she could. No father received more devoted and effective support from a beautiful and talented daughter. Jane Nevins as editor extraordinaire reminded me of the book's value whenever I flagged and guided me out of the many snarls and tangles I generated. I owe my deepest debt of gratitude to Jean McHugh—as ever my first discerning reader, whose thoughts, suggestions, and judgments, here as elsewhere, never fail to illuminate what I struggle to grasp. I'm indebted to her for so much, not least for her support while I wrestled with this project.

Critical were the contributions of my cardiologist, Stephen Achuff; my internist, Charles Angell; my surgeon, William Baumgartner; and my anesthetist, Daniel Nyhan. They carried me successfully through a bout of coronary insufficiency and bypass surgery smack in the middle of writing this book. Obviously, without their tireless efforts on my behalf none of this would have seen the light of day. My sincere—indeed heartfelt—thanks, gentlemen.

Introduction

What's wrong with psychiatry? For the better part of my career I have been asking myself and others this question about the profession that has been my life's work.

I ask it having repeatedly witnessed how faddish misdirections of thought and therapeutic practice sweep across the field to dominate opinion and action for years, only to sink from favor and fade away, leaving wounded patients and public scorn in their wake. One must wonder why psychiatrists learn so little from these misdirections, because they all follow the same pattern: seeing in human mental disorders things that do not exist, building treatment programs that are doomed, and then unapologetically retreating from these claims and therapies to await some other apparition to recapture the profession's loyalty and attention.

As an appalling example, in the early 1980s, a group of prominent psychiatrists claimed that certain mental symptoms indicated a past history of childhood sexual abuse in patients who insisted they had no memory of such experiences, and they alleged that these symptoms could be relieved if, and only if, the patients "recovered" their memories and dealt with them. Within the decade, this idea gained broad support not only from individual psychotherapists but also from such citadels of authority as academic psychiatric hospitals, psychiatry teaching departments, and even the National Institute of Mental Health in Bethesda. And yet the idea rested on claims unsupported by evidence, on speculation unrestrained by caution, and on the trust in authority that leads patients to accept suggestion. It vividly displayed the foundational vulnerabilities to mischief and misdirection that abides in psychiatric thought and practice.

I write about this episode now because it represents in almost pure form the kind of error that psychiatrists regularly fall into and thus has a clear message to teach. I was someone with a front-row seat in American academic psychiatry, who witnessed the injuries to people it exacted, and who, in protesting against it, came upon—as I had before—the power of this discipline to protect itself from criticism. I can tell the story from start to finish and believe that by describing it fully I can accomplish several useful objectives. Not only may I help prevent its repetition and mitigate the willingness of the public to accept such incoherence from psychotherapists, but I can explain just how proper psychiatric practice is carried out and what patients should expect from doctors and therapists as they strive to bring them the best treatments.

In this book, I will describe the calamitous course of the recovered memory movement in psychiatric practice and how the theories on which it was based proved invalid and pernicious. Eventually the public, to its amazement, came to realize that, with the procedures promoted by psychiatric "experts," a craze reminiscent of the Salem witch hunts had emerged from the psychiatric clinics. Several components, each of interest in itself, make up the story I plan to tell.

The first component describes some of the clinical incidents I encountered. They reveal what I learned from patients and their families as the idea of repressed memory emerged, promoted by a group of zealots so confident of their mission that they never questioned the dangerous and crude therapeutic practices they employed. I describe my part in the history, when—to the mortification of psychiatrists with any pride in their discipline—reform had to come not from the profession itself but from the civil government, which intervened to preserve social justice in the face of vicious abuse of authority and license.

(2.) The second component considers the long-term implications of this calamity for the psychiatric discipline. The most obvious effect is the general public's current distrust in the judgment and even the integrity of psychotherapists. This is not a trivial matter, given that people fearful of mistreatment may resist turning to the help they need. What constitutes proper and safe psychotherapeutic practices must be made clear again.

A subtle but momentous implication is the repressed memory movement's discrediting of Freudian psychoanalysis. A cozy niche for psychoanalysis was disrupted by the movement's disastrous misdirection, but as I shall strive to make clear, Freudianism regrouped, somewhat chastened, but just as determined to legitimize equally fallacious if not so crudely injurious views about mental disorders and their causes.

(3) The third and final component of the story deals with the practical questions that dawn on people after any disaster. These include questions of an immediate kind, such as where they or relatives can find services worthy of their trust and how they might protect themselves if another fad or mistreatment emerges in the future.

But more ultimate questions include considerations over how psychiatrists and other mental health workers who work under the auspices of a public license are being educated, what scientific traditions they depend upon, and whether psychiatric authorities are capable of adjudging standards of professional education and practice. The judicial system had to set them right on this occasion, but did anything change?

The story in this book is personal and tied to my experience as a psychiatric director who found himself in a fight he didn't seek, over matters of huge consequence to both the patients he was treating and the students he was teaching. I have written it because I want not only to record these events but also to emphasize how our success was another "nearest run thing," and to show how this history captures the larger and continuing problem of patients' vulnerability to psychiatric misdirection and incoherence.

The victory depended on several gifted and committed people whose scientific contributions turned the tide, and not a few plain but courageous individuals who were willing to suffer scorn and insults from the champions of recovered memory therapy (and from bystanders who should have known better) to get the truth of this terrible abuse of authority identified and corrected. All need to be remembered.

I have a final hope—that the description of just how psychiatrists ought to act and what they must avoid may dispel the aura of mystery and inscrutability that has emanated from the field for decades. This mystique certainly played some role in sustaining the misdirection by putting the ideas of psychiatrists beyond criticism as experts on the "mysteries of the mind."

People must relate to psychiatrists just as they do to other physicians. They should be able to grasp what psychiatrists can and cannot do by understanding what these doctors know and how they know it. Patients now understand the advice and treatment they receive at the hands of their physicians and surgeons in just such terms.

With this story in mind, perhaps everyone might agree that the time for psychiatrists to seek a similar understanding with the public and with their patients has arrived. This is the hope for the future that has spurred me to write this book.

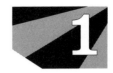

Meeting the Issue

A parable familiar to doctors speaks of a man rescuing people from a river—pulling them to safety as they splash helplessly past. He keeps at it: saving some, losing others, fighting the current, suffering the cold. At last he grasps what should have been obvious to him earlier and scrambles upstream to find out who's throwing these people in. There he discovers a tough gang and faces a new, more difficult challenge.

The parable fits my story. Over the course of eight months in 1990, I tussled with three incidents that I never fully grasped until I looked "upriver." There I found a group of psychiatrists producing my "downstream" experiences. Their practices and ideas—throwbacks, I thought, to discredited ways of the past—were gathering authority, taking on recruits, and dominating the rounds and conferences of many psychiatric educational programs. They were beginning to move into the public realms of civil and criminal law, where, like witch-hunters of old, they were threatening the defenseless and would ultimately shake public trust in psychiatry.

This discovery drew me into what was the biggest professional battle that I'd ever encountered over matters fraught with human meaning and supported by zealous and vocal advocates with whom I would have to quarrel. The quarrels would spill out of the hospital and my office, propelling me into courtrooms for testimony and distant legal offices for depositions, into surly confrontations in auditoriums and ugly professional exchanges in journals, into public attention and private miseries. Each of the three "downstream" events that drew my attention (and that I handled clumsily) has its own interesting story.

The first occurred in a nonclinical setting and without much fanfare. Baltimore's Hamilton Street Club is a genial luncheon and conversation club for men and women of some achievement in that city. The club's noon lunches gave me the chance to meet and talk with people working in fields other than medicine.

One afternoon in the spring of 1990, just before we went into the dining room, a member of the club took me aside to ask my professional advice. He recounted a strange tale. One evening a few days earlier, his niece, whom he hadn't seen for more than a decade because she lived in Washington State, appeared unannounced at his front door. Refusing to come in, she declared from the porch that she had crossed the country to confront him about events of long ago—his gross sexual abuse of her when she was a child.

The man was appalled by her charge. He repudiated the accusation, saying that he had never harmed her in any way but had always regarded her with family interest and affection. The young woman dismissed his response and refused to discuss any details of her claim that might clear things up; rather, parting from him promptly, she avowed that her memory was clear, that she carried permanent psychological burdens and scars from his abuse, and that she was not surprised by his denial of the events because she had been warned to expect it. She left him mystified and disturbed.

"Why would she make such weird claims?" he asked me. "I haven't seen her for years. Even when she was a youngster I didn't have that much to do with her, and I certainly never took advantage of her—or anyone else—as she's maintaining. She must be mixed up. But it's really disturbing, and I'm not sure what to do."

I said I couldn't say what could be troubling his niece but that several things came to mind. I told him I'd be happy to look into the matter if he wished. I thought she might be delusional and paranoid—psychotic with some illness or affected by some drug. Certainly she must have been in an unusual mental state—traveling across the country just to hurl venomous accusations from the doorstep at a relative she hadn't seen in years. But what specifically was wrong I couldn't say.

He was eager for me to explore the matter. Having seen his niece in such an agitated condition, he worried about what it meant for her and, of course, for him, given her charge.

I can't say that I dwelled much on the possibility that he was guilty of the offense (although, of course, I couldn't rule it out). He wasn't acting like someone in the wrong. If the charges were true—and he actually had sexually (and thus criminally) abused a minor some years before—then he'd be unlikely to broach the matter with an acquaintance in a semipublic setting or to ask that friend to inquire into the situation in ways that would draw more attention to it. A guilty man would surely have consulted a lawyer in private, or done nothing in hopes that his accuser would not press the matter.

I planned a simple response to his request. I would try to reach doctors who might know her, would describe her strange behavior here in Baltimore, the delusional character of her claims, and ask what was being done to help her. Such professional interactions are standard when mysterious behaviors are witnessed. They rest on the principle that diagnostic practice and protective treatments should derive from sound information.

I didn't believe that my inquiry could be construed as an invasion of the niece's medical privacy because, outside a clinical office, she was making public accusations with heavy implications. No one in Baltimore could know whether she might be planning even more destructive behavior.

My Hamilton Street Club acquaintance was able to get the name of his niece's psychiatrist in Washington State, and I had links to the Northwest because for two years, in 1973–75, I had been the chairman of the Psychiatry Department at the University of Oregon. Thus I found and called her physician one afternoon. Despite my explaining, through his secretary, our worries about the woman and our need for reassurance that she was under care, the doctor refused to talk about the case with me; he wouldn't even come to the phone.

Why did I think this was unusual? I'm aware that psychotherapists, when embarked on a course of therapy, will tell the patient that, during the therapy, no one else will be consulted. But usually before therapy starts doctors following the guidelines of common sense want to be certain that their plans rest on all the information available. In this way they can develop the best treatment for their patients and know all the implications—public and private—of taking on therapeutic responsibilities.

I had become accustomed—again because of what had become standard practice at Johns Hopkins—to work with doctors who were anxious to check their facts and presumptions. Did he know she'd made this trip east? Did he know of her claims about her uncle? Did he think them true or delusional? Did he not want to learn about the incident in Baltimore and the uncle's version of the past?

But this man didn't even get on the phone to say that he was confident of his diagnosis and was now treating the patient accordingly. He wouldn't even acknowledge this transcontinental trip, much less say whether it was at his instigation or an impulse of the patient. He wouldn't offer some reassurance that my friend, despite his niece's wild appearance, need not worry about her or himself.

When even that small help was not proffered, I had to think what to make of the situation. I concluded most unsatisfactorily that somehow I had stumbled across an anomalous situation—one in which the behaviors of both the patient and the clinician were in flux—and that I'd best leave my number and presume that, if matters worsened, I would hear before anything untoward happened to concern us in Baltimore.

And that's what I told my friend. He had been, I said, a victim of an aberrant practitioner struggling in a confused way with a difficult patient. I had seen such confusions work out with time in psychotherapy, especially if, after an honest, good faith effort to help, the situation was left alone. I told him that he would be unlikely to hear anything more from that quarter. And so it turned out.

His experience was over. My experience, however, was about to grow, and my presumptions about how psychiatry was practiced outside of Hopkins about to be shaken. From a distance of almost two decades, I mark this Hamilton Street Club encounter and the unease it awakened in me as my entry into psychiatry's civil war. I now think that the psychiatrist had induced the woman's belief in her abuse and had encouraged her to come to Baltimore and accuse her uncle, believing that it somehow might confirm the idea. He was not looking for a challenging call from me.

The second incident emerged soon after the first, during a set meeting I held with the resident physicians in my department. At these regular meetings, we discussed psychiatric research and practice, given that the residents were soon to venture forth on their own. One mentioned hearing about patients at the Sheppard and Enoch Pratt Hospital, a renowned private psychiatric hospital just outside Baltimore's city limits, who claimed to have dual or multiple personalities. Dr. Richard Loewenstein, he said, had recently moved to Baltimore from California and, on starting an inpatient service for multiple personality disorder (MPD) at Sheppard, had stirred up some attention. The resident wondered what I thought about the matter given that MPD is vanishingly rare.

I'd seen a few patients claiming to have several personalities, but they had emerged shortly after the book and movie *The Three Faces of Eve* had depicted a case of MPD back in the late 1950s. Those patients seemed to have picked up hints from the film and were imitating the character of Eve portrayed so vividly by the actress Joanne Woodward.

The textbook of psychiatry I used in England during my education there had been explicit: "It seems that these multiple personalities are always artificial productions, the product of the medical attention (and also literary interest) that they arouse."[1] I'd successfully treated those few patients I'd seen by turning attention away from the display and toward their more everyday problems of depression and discouragement.

I therefore taught that MPD fell into the broad range of human behavior disorders that psychiatrists had in the past termed hysteria or hysterical.

By the term *hysteria* and its adjective *hysterical*, psychiatrists did not mean wildly emotional or hyperdramatic, although some patients may have had such features of temperament. Rather they meant behaviors that mimic debilitating disease or disorder and have the effect of drawing medical attention, consuming medical resources, and masking or exaggerating more straightforward clinical issues.

My residents, though, had never seen an MPD patient during their years of clinical experience and were naturally curious about them. They asked whether we might invite Dr. Loewenstein to visit with us and present his work.

I was happy to agree and looked forward to the meeting, expecting to encounter a student of this condition who could explore with us this domain by perhaps showing us a patient and reviewing the odd phasic history of the disorder (extending back to the nineteenth century), in which, like some style of dress or fashion, it periodically sprang up and then disappeared from among psychiatric patients. How differently it all turned out.

The day arrived, and Dr. Loewenstein stood before us. He was a trimly bearded man of modest stature who wore metal frame glasses, dressed in a neatly tailored suit, and carried himself with that air of self-assurance that I'm afraid I'd seen before in psychiatrists who believed they could impart some deep secret about humankind.

We three dozen or so Hopkins psychiatrists were told by him that, contrary to what we thought, multiple personality disorder occurred frequently and that we were probably missing it on a regular basis. In fact, he found MPD quite often in patients who had seen several other psychiatrists who had not even dreamed of that diagnostic possibility.

He went on to describe how doctors needed to be "active" in eliciting the alternative personalities ("alters" he called them). Hypnosis was one of the active methods he used to gain the confidence of patients and draw forth the alters. Other methods were more in the form of relaxation techniques, often enhanced by sedatives, that took the form of guiding the patients into trancelike states where alters could be called forth.

He told us how he probed with questions such as "Have you ever felt like another part of you does things that you can't control?" If the patient gave ambiguous answers, he dug further along these lines, striving to get the patient to describe feelings of being "sort of disconnected" in some setting, such as while driving for a distance or during routines that do not demand full attention. Then he sought to learn of any shifts in mood or thought that would hint at some splitting away from the scene in ways suggesting to him the emergence of "another" personality. If he could get patients to agree that there is something like another "part" to their personality, then he often would press the issue by asking quite directly, "Does this part have a name?"

In these ways, he told us, he had frequently surprised onlookers (and at first even himself) when the patients produced some name that, when tied to a particular set of characteristics (age, sex, skills, temperament, and memories), satisfied, as he said, "the operational diagnostic criteria" for MPD.

After he described these techniques, along with several anecdotes of patient responses, Dr. Loewenstein brought his talk to a conclusion with an idea that—given the suggestion-laden way he approached patients—did not actually surprise me. My previous experience with psychoanalysts and their teachings about the workings of the "unconscious" had prepared me for what he was to say. MPD, he said, was the manifestation in the conscious mind of the destruction of its integrity by childhood sexual abuse—an abuse so severe and unsuitable that it often was driven from conscious memory by the mind's defensive mechanisms of "repression" or, as he preferred, "dissociation."

Every one of the patients with MPD, identified by the methods he described, had been assaulted by a trusted and beloved person during childhood. Prior to his treatment, they were "unaware" of the events, because they were "unbearable" both as physical and psychological traumas and in terms of the ugly implications they carried about trusted members of the family. This "secret" had been carried in the unconscious by the patient from the time of the abuse, and it represented the "germ" or "hidden defect" at the heart of the patient's presenting mental difficulties—whether those difficulties were anxiety states, depression, marital difficulties, or the like.

MPD emerged because the maneuvers of repression/dissociation hid the trauma from consciousness but at the expense of a smooth and unified development of mental life and mental faculties. As a result of sequestering from consciousness these thoughts, memories, and feelings, the patient could not subsequently experience mental life as an integrated stream of faculties and functions. Rather it was experienced as broken into disconnected, partially inaccessible, distinct clusterings of thoughts, feelings, and responses best captured by the term "alternate personalities."

Some alter clusterings, he posited, held the memories of the trauma that were inaccessible to other alter clusterings that carried out the ordinary daily life of the patient. Psychiatrists could first reach these hidden alters by hypnotizing the "host" personality and then having the alters describe the traumatic experiences.

The patients lived with these features of mind from childhood and thought of them as "normal." They would, however, reveal these characteristics of their shattered mental lives to those, such as Dr. Loewenstein and members of his staff, who knew how to piece together equivocal and partial answers and press the patients toward honest and complete replies.

Only people ready to provide unequivocal support for these patients should carry out such work, we were told, because as the patients abandoned the unsatisfactory MPD mode of keeping the "secret," they would realize and experience in full consciousness the misery of the sexual betrayal they suffered as children.

Dr. Loewenstein presented these opinions as though they were indisputable. He believed that, at least in his hands, the methods to draw out the patients were so dependable that they would never generate false examples. He also held that the source of MPD in childhood abuse could not be doubted—in part because of the testimony from the patients and in part because it "made sense" of the disorder. He was sure that many MPD patients were to be found on our wards and clinics but that we were overlooking them—to their detriment—because we were not using his methods or thinking his way. He tied it all together plausibly and with confidence.

I found his presentation far from compelling. We had heard an opinion without any means to test it. We heard of no efforts to confirm the presumptions of child abuse outside of patient testimony. We saw no patient we might question, he told of no efforts to study rates of diagnostic error, we saw neither long-term results of treatment nor any assessment of the costs and psychological burdens these treatments might carry.

I believed that Dr. Loewenstein and his group were manufacturing MPD rather than discerning or detecting it. In this sense MPD was an artifact inadvertently produced by them during their assessment and not a product of nature revealed to them by that assessment. Specifically, I thought it likely that they caused trusting and vulnerable patients to respond with "alters" by leading them—under hypnosis and with sedation—into manifesting the assumptions the therapists held and behaviors they expected.

I could not be sure of my suspicions given what we heard, but I did know that a similar psychiatric misdirection produced clinical artifacts in the late nineteenth century. A renowned French physician, Jean-Martin Charcot, treated patients at La Salpêtrière Hospital in Paris in ways very like Dr. Loewenstein and his group appeared to be doing at Shephard.

In Paris, patients with emotional disorders were housed on the same wards as patients with epilepsy. Charcot, a leading figure in Parisian medicine and society, was attentive to the epileptics and failed at first to recognize that the emotionally disturbed patients on the ward were imitating them. Charcot came to believe that these patients must have some new disease—"hystero-epilepsy," he called it—and the patients, trusting that important facts were being discovered, cooperated with Charcot by reproducing these symptoms on his command. He began to show the patients as examples of a newly discovered condition at his Thursday public teaching round.

It was only after patients began to become more and more disruptive that one of his students, Joseph Babinski, pointed out that if the doctors stopped calling attention to symptoms, the patients gradually stopped exhibiting them. He realized that the ward environment, the doctor's attention, and the patients' search for help all could combine to promote behaviors that could be difficult to differentiate from illness.

When, with this example in mind, I questioned Dr. Loewenstein about the possibility of suggestion and social contagion on his services, he asked me whether I had any "data" to support my ideas. "Data?" I replied. "You're the one making the claim of a new discovery, so you're the one to supply the data. I'm challenging your claim by calling attention to another explanation

13

for the phenomena you're describing. It's for you to do the defending by bringing forth pertinent observations ('data' if you will) that would answer the challenge."

Our rather academic but slightly heated exchange over roles and responsibilities continued for a few minutes without being resolved. After a few questions from other members of the audience, the meeting broke up.

I stayed mildly irritated but thought that I may have conveyed a point to my students and other members of the department about how clinical reasoning worked and how the burden of proof is carried by the proponents of a new idea. I now realize that I was too preoccupied with my teaching role and overlooked what this lecture did herald. Still "downstream" in my thoughts and actions, I failed to ask whether these ideas were growing or to wonder how many patients were being misled. I began my voyage upstream after incident three.

I met Richard Moore when we served together on the board of a nonprofit group in Baltimore. A tall, handsome ex–naval officer, he offered analysis and guidance to an organization that badly needed help. I subsequently ran into him and his wife, Jane, in other contexts and found them a gracious pair. When they asked to see me one day, I was happy to oblige.

It turned out that their daughter, married and independent, had fallen into a severe depression and was being seen at Sheppard Pratt Hospital. Her social worker had called asking them to come to the hospital for a meeting to discuss "things." The Moores wanted to know why I thought they would be called, given that their daughter was married, that she was rather touchy about her independence from them, and that her own husband had not asked for or was even aware of this proposal from the social worker.

I drew no link to Dr. Loewenstein—Sheppard is a large psychiatric hospital—and thought the matter was a straightforward clinical inquiry. I told them that the social worker probably wanted to gather more information about their daughter's family history, personality, educational experience, and the like so as to enhance the hospital's treatment plans. This was not her first attack of depression, and more information might improve her future. We do this often at Hopkins, I told them, and assured them that it would not be unpleasant.

I was a bit perplexed, though, that the doctors hadn't already told them what to expect and how family meetings can help diagnostic efforts. I should have worried more about that thought, and perhaps I'd have aided them if I'd been more alert to the times and called the hospital myself to clarify the purpose of this family visit.

But following my reassurance, the Moores went and were ushered into a room with their daughter, the social worker, and the doctor. Without a preamble beyond introductions, the social worker told Richard that they had learned from their daughter that Richard had repeatedly sexually abused her when she was a small child and that Jane must have known and tolerated his behavior.

No proof for these claims was offered. But she thought the Moores might "acknowledge these facts" and prepare to help the hospital treatment team heal their daughter's psychological injuries. The Moores were outraged by these accusations, however, and after protesting to everyone in the room to no avail, decided to leave and think over what was best to do for their daughter and each other.

Still reeling from what she saw now as a kind of professional ambush, Jane called me that afternoon to recount what had transpired and how her husband and she had rejected the charges. She told me that while their family, like most, had strenuous periods, mostly tied to the demands of Richard's military service and professional life, they took them in stride and weathered them, so she thought, unscathed.

She protested that Richard was ever a devoted father who would never think of abusing his or any other child. Jane, who knew his comings and goings throughout the household, never saw anything that would prompt a suspicion in her, a most intelligent and conscientious mother, hardly one who would surrender her children to vicious tyranny.

On hearing of this incident, I decided to visit Sheppard Pratt and discuss what evidence had prompted the staff's opinions about the Moores and led to this ambush-like family forum. I was still "downstream," presuming that I was dealing with a random incident rather than a group "upstream" ganging up on people and producing victims. I thought more information about the persons I knew would either clear up a mistake or prove I was wrong to trust them. The doctor and the social worker agreed to meet me at the doctor's private office in suburban Towson.

I asked them for the evidence on which they built their conclusions that their patient had been sexually abused, that Richard was an incestuous pedophile, and that Jane was a yielding accomplice. They looked at me as if my questions didn't make sense.

"You're searching for the equivalent of an X-ray," the doctor said. "But we have the revealing mental state of this woman." Like Loewenstein, the doctor went on to argue, as though it had been firmly established, that children quite commonly forget all about sexual abuse for years only to have aspects of the forgotten memories surface in adulthood in the form of otherwise inexplicable depressions, anxieties, or spousal discord. The confrontation with the Moores, they said, was part of the therapy: getting the "truth" out in the open so the patient could begin to "heal."

I tried to shake the doctor and the social worker out of their beliefs. I noted how nothing of this sort had ever been claimed by the patient when treated before at their hospital for depression, and nothing about Richard indicated that he had sexual hang-ups. This vigorous, busy, friendly man was hardly the type to prey on small children. He and his wife had enjoyed a long and companionable marriage that left her with no fears about his nature.

The doctor and the social worker simply dismissed these views of mine with clichés such as "Things like this happen in the best of families." They provided me with no more evidence for the abuse than the patient's presenting depressive symptoms and her willingness now to "acknowledge" the abuse with their "treatment." They made themselves out as staunch defenders of "the victim" and me out as the craven advocate for "the perpetrators."

Our session lasted little more than ten minutes before the doctor noted that I was "too biased to be reasonable." I was ushered out as someone "knowledgeable professionals" could not and should not argue with.

I was now cross and much more frustrated than I had been by Dr. Loewenstein's presentation. I had misled the Moores with my reassurance, encouraged them to trust psychiatrists and so to walk into an ambush. I felt

I had to take some action on behalf of Richard, document that this man was innocent, and find some proof that would convince everyone that he did not abuse children—evidence beyond his word and that of his wife.

I proposed that he take a polygraph lie-detector test to answer the accusations. Although these tests are not infallible, if he was willing to undergo the ordeal, the results would strengthen (or shake) my presumption of his innocence.

Moore was ready—eager indeed—for the test. I was able to arrange for a polygraph expert from Langley, Virginia, to come to Baltimore and conduct it.

But before proceeding any further in a situation that was seemingly worsened by every action I took, I decided to consult with a psychiatrist I knew in Philadelphia, Dr. Martin Orne. I had good reasons for making this call.

Dr. Orne was a man who had done world-class scientific work on modes of psychological influence and control, with special emphasis on hypnosis and other forms of suggestion. He was a recognized genius at designing psychological investigations and experiments that dispelled psychiatric mysteries. Since Dr. Loewenstein told us that hypnosis was used at Sheppard to "recover" memories of childhood abuse and to discover "alters" in MPD, I expected that Orne was more advanced than I on these phenomena and their contemporary expressions.

He was also an experienced, thoughtful clinician and an approachable, coherent colleague. He knew how clinicians can go wrong and just how difficult it often was then to reason with them. And he had seen the coming and going of all the fads that I had seen and more besides, given his acquaintance with the world of hypnosis, cults, nontraditional healings, and the like. Clinical skill, brilliant gifts, extensive knowledge, broad experimental experience wrapped in a friendly courteous warm exterior were just what I needed. Perhaps he could advise me in this situation.

This decision marked my belated turn "upstream" to discover at last what I was facing and what all three downstream incidents actually represented.

From his office at the University of Pennsylvania, Orne responded to my question about my plans for a polygraph examination.

"Absolutely press ahead. It does put the accused at risk, but his willingness to accept the risk without demurring is to his credit. Although the procedure is humiliating, you both face the awkward circumstance of having to "prove a negative" [i.e., demonstrate years after an alleged event that it did *not* happen]. A properly carried out polygraph that the subject passes indicates that he is in no doubt that he is telling the truth in the face of these charges. It's the best first step in restoring family confidence and reassuring critics that you have taken the accusations seriously."

Then he added. "I'm sure he'll pass this test but call me again after it's over. I can tell you a good bit more about what you're facing and what's happening here in Philadelphia."

With that advice I pressed ahead, and the grim day when Richard was polygraphed arrived. He sat in a chair in my office at Hopkins stripped to the waist, hooked up to the polygraph machine. He looked strong, confident, tough—and he went on to pass the test without a tremor—but I felt sickened by the sight of this first-rate person undergoing this degrading process. Had we really reached the point in psychiatry where this was necessary?

I called Martin Orne the next day to tell him the good results. He and I agreed that I should inform the daughter's doctor and social worker—but he predicted (again accurately) that the information would not shake their opinions.

In fact, and quite sadly, nothing seemed to shake the beliefs of the therapists (or now the daughter) that Richard had abused her in childhood. Since the events recounted, the Moore family has remained distressfully estranged. Mr. and Mrs. Moore have reconciled themselves to this grim state of affairs but continue to hope that their daughter will come to realize that the real abusers of her were overenthusiastic, theory-driven therapists who misdirected her treatment.

For me this last episode was the "wake up" event. I had stumbled badly and led some good people into trouble. It prompted further conversations with Martin Orne, who explained that what I had encountered was not strange to him. He described how he first heard of psychiatrists and psychologists pushing the use of hypnosis as a means of "recovering" memories and realized how misguided they were about hypnosis and the validity of claims that rested upon it.

Most recently, he said, cases of "recovered memories" along with MPD were turning up in Philadelphia. A couple of the more distinguished hospitals (the Institute of the Pennsylvania Hospital and Friends Hospital) had treatment programs identical to that at Sheppard. He had been drawn into helping several families all of whom faced allegations similar to those confronted by the Moores.

"I believe it's happening all over the country and you've just seen the beginnings of it in Baltimore," he said. And he was absolutely right. I had failed to see—until hit hard by case examples—that members of my discipline had relapsed into disputed ways of thinking about mental illness, similar to but much cruder than standard Freudian psychoanalysis. The practices these ways of thinking supported would prove very difficult to interrupt and would produce much damage to patients, families, and the psychiatric profession before they were discredited.

I eventually came to learn the history behind these events. Childhood sexual abuse and multiple personality disorder were knotted together in 1973 by a strange, off-beat psychiatrist, Cornelia Wilbur. That year her ideas emerged in a best-selling paperback book entitled *Sybil* written for her by a journalist, Flora Rheta Schreiber.

This book might have provoked a transient uptick of interest in MPD, as had *The Three Faces of Eve*. But by claiming child abuse as the cause, it struck several arousing chords. It fit with the concerns of the times and it hooked in psychiatrists ever keen to explain mental illness by hidden sexual events.

Wilbur was trained in Freudian psychoanalysis and in the book describes her efforts to provide psychoanalytically informed treatment to a young woman with a crippling form of anxiety. The patient presented different moods on different days to Dr. Wilbur, who concluded that she, like Eve in *The Three Faces of Eve*, had the rare disorder MPD.

During the several years of therapy that followed, and with the help of hypnosis and barbiturate sedatives, Dr. Wilbur drew personalities from Sybil—she eventually "found" sixteen—and became convinced that the patient had been sexually abused by her mentally ill mother as a child. Her

Freudian-derived interest in the power of the unconscious and in sexual conflicts led her to this conviction. She drew the patient to this belief by interpreting every "alter" as isolating the painful memories from consciousness by splitting them off from the main ("host") personality.

Dr. Wilbur then assumed, on the basis of this case, that all the previously reported patients with MPD had been abused cruelly as children and that the abuse was most usually of a sexual kind. She began to find MPD patients regularly in her practice, as would the psychiatrists who followed after her. (In fact, they produced a diagnostic epidemic of thousands of patients. By 1986 Dr. Frank Putnam, a follower of Wilbur and a psychiatrist at the National Institutes of Health, could announce proudly that "more cases of MPD have been reported in the last 5 years than in the preceding two centuries.")

Wilbur and writer Flora Rheta Schreiber produced *Sybil* as a popular book vivid in anecdote because Wilbur could not succeed in getting her views published in reputable journals. At any other time in history the book's sentimental style and wild theories would have condemned it, but not in the America of 1973. It sold millions of copies (and became a TV movie, with Sally Field as the star patient, in 1976).

For the book and film *Sybil* appeared at a propitious time. Freudian psychoanalysis was fading as an attractive enterprise for many therapists. It had become an intellectual thicket where controversies of a scholastic kind divided the analysts into camps. It demanded large amounts of time and money from both trainees and patients (years of daily hour-long sessions, each costing hundreds of dollars). But most tellingly, its concepts of the divided self battling an internal war between instincts and civilization demanded patience and subtle thought for their study and didn't fit the fashions of the times or the educational background of the therapists now being trained in large numbers outside medicine and psychiatry. Simple explanations involving villains, victims, and foundational viciousness would thrive in these new times and with these new therapists.

Still many of the conceptual presumptions of psychoanalysis about how the mind works had become idiomatic among therapists. Ideas such as the conflict-ridden unconscious, sex and sexuality as the source of those conflicts, and repression hiding life's truths from patients were the currency of service in psychotherapeutic clinics.

These Freudian presumptions were easily co-opted and simply given new contents to serve the times. And so what I've called the Manneristic Freudians were born. They picked up Sybil, multiple personality, and shameful buried traumas from Cornelia Wilbur. They threw in repression, symptom formation, and psychic defenses. They ended by explaining mental disorders in a way that seemed at once fashionable and linked to tradition. Such a diagnostic regimen demanded little more than a high level of suspicion and a low level of skepticism.

Although an ordinary person might ask such questions as "Why 'multiple' personalities when just one 'extra' would serve?" or "Why didn't Eve's psychiatrists find abuse?" the Mannerists drew followers from the throngs of therapists looking for a novel up-to-date program. They had to be drawn by the magic of these themes because no clinical trials or follow-up studies were offered in support of related treatments. Just when I was first encountering this issue, Dr. Frank Putnam, although writing a book about how to diagnose and treat MPD, admitted that "lack of outcome data is both surprising and dismaying. ... There are only a few professional articles together with a number of novelized or autobiographical accounts of treatment, that hint at a favorable outcome."[2]

This was not going to change. Assumptions, expectations, even fantasies would promote and sustain the phenomena I was encountering. The psychiatric journals did nothing to interrupt what their editors believed was a kindly intended treatment for traumatically abused people and thus beyond criticism. This failure of professional oversight would eventually turn into a huge embarrassment for psychiatry.

At the time of my first "downstream" encounters, none of this was as clear as it would become. But I did finally move "upstream" and into a battle over the most fundamental matters of my field.

In fact, this battle would call upon skills I had practiced and assumptions I had drawn from the start of my psychiatric education. By dramatically demonstrating how psychiatry was riven by factions, it would re-call not only the concepts and methods I learned from my earliest teachers but also their admonitions and prophesies. It is to how I had been readied for such a clash (even though I had not anticipated it) that I turn in the next chapter.

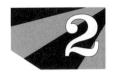

The Path
Less Traveled

An important aspect of this story relates to how my criticisms and opposition to the recovered memory disaster grew from my early medical education when I first began to approach psychiatric thought and practice. During my years as a student, intern, and resident at the Harvard Medical School in the 1950s, I was introduced to and ultimately directed away from the Freudian school of psychiatry. The experience would immunize me against the kind of sweeping and speculative concepts about the human mind and its workings that promoted an embrace of such novelties as "recovered memories."

In the 1950s, though, Freudian psychoanalysis was the dominant explanatory theory in American psychiatry and was particularly strong at Harvard when I was a medical student. It was deemed the most coherent theory of the functioning of the human mind and one that offered the clearest explanations of mental disorders. It also furnished the foundation for an approach to treating mental disorders by drawing out hidden thoughts and feelings of the patients in psychotherapy.

Long-standing therapeutic approaches to psychiatric disorders, such as viewing them as reactions to life circumstances and treating them as forms of exhaustion and breakdown, were dismissed by my Freudian teachers as superficial, insignificant, and useless. Although a similar criticism of "no evidence" could at the time be said of the Freudian treatments—no obvious cures were demonstrated—the promise of enlightenment embedded in the Freudian theories attracted followers from among the best and brightest of my medical school friends, who encouraged me to join them.

Boston, town and gown, had taken to Freudian psychology and psychotherapy like a religious awakening. Especially for young men and women, Freudian ideas seemed to explain so much about human nature and to suggest even more about the reforming of society that an enthusiasm of almost Salvationist hope carried them along. They read Freudian texts, interpreted every thought of themselves and others in Freudian terms, and were all either in or thinking of getting into Freudian psychotherapy usually for treatment for their youth-related heartaches as well as for initiation in the mysteries of the cult.

At first blush it might seem incredible that this city of legendary common sense and careful finance would so surrender to what amounts to an untested, romantic, and—as I'll describe—subversive theory. But even a modest knowledge of Boston's intellectual history reveals a long-standing susceptibility of its citizens to cultic absorptions over mind/matter theories, especially when tied to cures and curing. There stands the Mother Church for Christian Science as a monument to the countercultural movement of thought about bodily health and the power of spirituality launched from Boston in the nineteenth century. Also, as telling in its own way, Henry James's great novel *The Bostonians* describes the commitment to and authority of a "mesmeric healer" in Boston in the 1870s, suggesting that the secular and scientific fad of mesmerism, based on Franz Anton Mesmer's theories, had survived in Boston despite being discredited—as based on "imagination"—a hundred years previously, at its source in Paris, by a scientific commission that included Benjamin Franklin.

On reflection I've wondered whether Boston culture, zealous for fighting oppression since its glory days with abolition and inspired by Emerson's optimism, environmentalism, and Transcendentalist devotion to the intuitive, welcomed Freudian theory uncritically because it identified, as I'll describe, psychiatric disorders as products of social and family tyranny. And so at the Harvard Medical School in the 1950s (and for a couple of decades afterward) Freudian psychoanalysis was given a free rein, though it obviously created a schism between the ideas conveyed in psychiatry and the coherent messages of science that all other students of medicine and surgery were being taught to follow.

Specifically, at Harvard our psychiatric teachers, following Freud, told us that human consciousness, with its intentions, attitudes, and assumptions, was forged primarily by the psychic unrest within the "unconscious" generated by the "unavoidable" clash between the selfish, pleasure-seeking desires of infants and the demands of society for their conformity and restraint. From their picture of infant mental life as an encounter with the masked forces of social oppression within family life and thus as a tumult of conflicts and desires, our teachers derived all those familiar Freudian concepts of the Oedipus complex, castration fears, penis envy, and so forth.

We medical students learned that the unconscious residues of these formative conflicts, expressing themselves in "unguarded moments," such as during dreams and slips of the tongue, were at the root of psychiatric illnesses. And these disorders, they claimed, would succumb to therapists who could help patients bring to the light of consciousness their repressed but influential conflicts with social authority. They were to be guided into seeing that their relationships with their parents, especially the parent of the opposite sex, were fraught with sexual implications "repressed into the unconscious." If these repressed feelings could be brought to consciousness, these patients would not only deal more coherently with their life plans and interpersonal relations but also find relief from the symptomatic manifestations that brought them to the clinic.

We learned that the patients were encouraged to grasp these remarkable ideas by engaging in repeated sessions with psychoanalysts who had them rest on a couch and talk without restraint ("free associate") about their earlier life. The analyst subtly directed the sessions by showing approval and disapproval and in this way—usually over months or even years—won the

25

assent of the patient to Freudian assumptions that the presenting difficulties in one way or another represented the residual effects of the unresolved, psychologically buried conflicts over sexual—indeed incestuous—desires.

Behind all this teaching about mental disorder, and adding much to the appeal to us idealistic students, our instructors also claimed that Freud's ideas about how humans think and develop would, if broadly understood and translated into child rearing, education, and social action, transform our civilization for the better. By proclaiming that the ostensibly benevolent family was actually a site of human domination, deprivation, and hidden duplicities, psychoanalysis came to rival Marxism as a liberating ideology. It gained wide appeal outside of medicine and, as I noted earlier, struck a responsive chord in "abolitionist" Boston.

Only a few hardy souls were challenging these ideas in Boston, where my education continued at the Harvard-affiliated Peter Bent Brigham Hospital. By good fortune one of them addressed my then typical assumptions about psychiatry and its direction.

George Thorn was the Physician-in-Chief at the Brigham and took most seriously his responsibility for the educational development of all his medical interns. He was an accomplished and far-seeing medical scientist. He was the first person at Harvard to say that my plans for entering psychiatric training after internship were "incoherent" and needed to be reconsidered. In a series of meetings with me he argued that contemporary psychiatric training at Harvard, with its Freudian emphasis, was "a dead-end." He had come to this conclusion by noting the loss of personal growth in previous interns who had followed that path. "They become single-minded people," he warned me, "strangely self-preoccupied, learning nothing about the medical sciences that are growing all around us and in particular nothing about the brain and its role in mental life and its disorders. I don't see any future in that pathway and can't encourage my house officers to follow it."

His recommendation was that I chart a course different from what was standard with Harvard psychiatry but that with his and others' help would bring me into psychiatry via an immersion in neurology, where patients with brain disorders were studied and treated. "This," he assured me, "will give you a better foundation and bring to your attention important work about the brain that will soon be emerging of interest to any psychiatric clinician and investigator."

Dr. Thorn's proposal was defiantly contrary to everything that I had learned as a Harvard medical student. It had the appealing merit of providing an adventurous and unique career plan. And it put me ultimately in the hands of a most thorough teacher of medical thought and practice, Dr. Raymond Adams, the chief of the Neurology Department at the Massachusetts General Hospital, who accepted me into his program because of Dr. Thorn's recommendation and where I worked as a resident for three years.

Right from the start, Dr. Adams instilled in me confidence that this redirection of my career trajectory was on target. He did so by revealing just how contemporary medicine and neurology advanced as clinical disciplines and how psychoanalytic thought and practice were hindering psychiatry.

The issue turned simply on the methods neurologists and internists used to make sense of their patients and their clinical conditions. These methods were strikingly different from how psychoanalysts drew their opinions about patients. Whereas neurologists teach their students to work inductively, drawing their conclusions only after collecting a broad array of comprehensible and accessible data, psychoanalytic teaching encourages students to work deductively from theoretical presumptions, Freudian suppositions, and particular—ostensibly key—symptomatic presentations.

Again, because in practice psychoanalysts are sure that patients' problems rest upon some hidden sexual conflict, they turn every manifestation of distress, such as depression or anxiety, into proof of their views. Since all people have a sexual side to their lives, one can always find some event, attitude, or concern in that domain on which to build a case. The analysts "know" what to look for as soon as the patients describe their symptoms. They then press their deductions on the patients in the therapy that follows.

Specifically, as a deductive rather than inductive approach, psychoanalysts believe that Freud's presumptions about human mental life have such a self-evident character that they can use them to explain psychological symptoms in the same way Euclid worked deductively from self-evident axioms such as "a straight line can be drawn joining any two points" to solve geometry problems. As a result, psychoanalysts make clinical claims such as "hysterical behaviors derive from Oedipal conflicts" or "rigorous toilet training during infancy generates obsessional traits" and have such confidence in the logic of these claims that they can ignore counter opinions derived in more empirical inductive ways.

Dr. Adams and his associates had problems with these axiomatic presumptions not because they could not conceive them and certainly not because, as analysts like to assert, they were unwilling to accept "the complexity, depth, and darkness of human life,"[1] but because they did not see objective evidence for them. Dr. Adams taught that knowing how the mind works both normally and when symptom-ridden should comprise the goal rather than the starting place of clinicians.

Therefore, in contrast to psychoanalysts drawing upon preconceptions, contemporary physicians strive to begin their assessment with patients simply as they present in the clinic. Doctors work "up" from there by making use of all kinds of accessible observations—some about the patient, his or her presenting physical and mental state, and the onset and course of illness; some from reports of other people who know the patient and have watched the illness appear and progress; and some from laboratory data that, for example, display the image of the patient's brain for study.

From such a collection of reports, observations, and facts they strive to synthesize a diagnostic conception that identifies how and where the patient's body or brain was injured and how that kind of injury in precisely that region would likely produce the specific symptoms and signs of illness that the patient displays. In this synthetic process they will employ established knowledge about bodily and psychological functioning derived from the sciences that surround the discipline, such as neuroanatomy, physiology, brain pathology, or psychology. (Parenthetically, many of them become interested in and ultimately contribute to these sciences, having witnessed what they bring to bedside service.) Their interpretive opinion grows more confident with information but is ever open to challenge and correction if a new observation—an "ugly little fact"—comes to light that is incompatible with it.

This is the inductive or "scientific" method. It depends on observational skills (such as how to examine the body and the conscious mind), on technical knowledge (such as that provided by physiology and psychology), and on interpretive skills (such as the weighing of evidence and the consideration of alternatives). These are all employed in reaching probabilistic diagnostic conclusions that remain open to refinement, corroboration, or refutation. Rather than following a Euclidian model, physicians struggle to answer medical questions in the same way that scientists since Galileo have struggled with physics questions. Certainly, as my teachers made vividly clear, this approach has steadily—even exponentially—advanced the knowledge and skills of physicians and surgeons in the last century.

In recounting these principles, Dr. Adams and my other instructors at the Massachusetts General Hospital drew several subtle implications about doctoring and human nature—implications that at first seemed to me trivial and petty but turned out to be portents of what transpired in the psychiatric controversies I later worked through. Their key point was that a deductive as opposed to inductive stance has a far-reaching effect on a practitioner's mind-set, most evident when directing treatments or responding to challenges.

Practitioners like psychoanalysts committed to the deductive development of their opinions from axiomatic, fixed premises about how the mind works will tend to acquire a self-assertive way of steering treatments along doctrinaire paths. They customarily reject criticisms of their views by scornfully suggesting some kind of "bad faith" at the root of every challenge ("Freud bashers" is a favorite rejoinder to critics of psychoanalysis), and be undeterred by poor outcomes, explaining them away as "expected" in the course of the therapy "yet to be completed."

Certainly with Freud as their exemplar, psychoanalysts have been quick to propose either bias or ignorance in their critics. They have such confidence in their axioms and their deductive judgments that they presume that challenges to their practices must be irrational and probably depend upon some neurotic, defensive response in the critic against the "revelations" of psychoanalysis. (This self-confident practice with deductive judgments also explains why psychoanalysts too often give voice to impertinent or hostile interpretations of colleagues and acquaintances in nonclinical settings—an ugly aspect of their culture.)

For similar reasons, psychoanalysts have proved indifferent supporters of psychiatric research. Given their trust in deductive conclusions, they see empirical investigation as but a tedious effort to prove what is obvious. They even suggest that practices based on an empirical approach can lead to an arid, faceless, and uninspired psychiatry.

Doctors using the inductive approach can, of course, become overconfident and go wrong. Their errors include using shortcuts to their conclusions, overvaluing some observations, and skipping crucial steps. (Sir William Osler, arguably the last century's first and finest teacher of physicians, memorably said, "The chief function of the consultant is to make the rectal examination you omitted").

Doctors learn early (sometimes from their patient's autopsy!) that success in inductive reasoning depends on having all the pertinent information. They usually respond to a challenge by considering its substance rather than addressing the personality or supposed agenda of its proponent. (Again William Osler: "One is never very surprised or angry to find that one's opponents are in the right.")[2] Also, an inductive stance naturally supports scientific investigation, since better knowledge and new discoveries augment interpretive power.

And finally to the idea that the science-bred inductive approach might lead to an uninspired and technical psychiatry—with neglect of the art and humane spirit of medicine—I thought my teachers offered the most telling answers. They noted that patients want doctors to be effective, to bring them cures, but then to get out of their lives. The quickest way to those goals was the method they were teaching. Their subtext was that doctors are not to use patients for self-fulfillment by enlisting them in social movements or rebellion. This is a gross misuse of medical privilege.

They went even further in telling me what to expect about my own career if I followed their path. If, they said, psychiatry moved as a discipline away from accepting sweeping new conjectures about how the mind functions and falters, then all psychiatric work—both clinical practice and research—would become much more exacting *and* much less dramatic. No longer would enthusiasm for "A Great Leader"—some Freud, Jung, or Adler—sweep the discipline. Rather, progress would depend on the slow, collaborative, and mutually supportive efforts of many patient toilers whose attitudes toward each other would depend solely on what each contributed.

In one way or another they told me that it was time for everyone interested in the study and treatment of mental disorders to grow up. "Stop thinking in visionary terms and accept a life like ours," they admonished. This life was, they described, characterized by much plodding effort made agreeable by the soundness of one's achievements, a sense of progress, and the satisfactions of scientifically broadened horizons from which new discoveries could be anticipated.

And so it proved. Nothing earth-shattering emerged from what seemed then to my friends in psychiatry the maverick path I elected to follow. But I and those who came to join me can point to a sizable number of achievements all derived from emphasizing three fundamentally scientific practices in our teaching and our work: careful observations, systematic measurements, and the employment in psychiatry of the same inductive method that works in neurology and other forms of medicine.

Even more of this approach was taught to me at the Institute of Psychiatry in London, where, after my three years at the Massachusetts General Hospital Neurology Department, I studied under the direction of Sir Aubrey Lewis and was closely supervised by future British professors of psychiatry James Gibbons and Gerald Russell. They had followed the same path from neurology into psychiatry and were familiar with the application of the scientific method to psychiatric patients.

Again it depends on gathering information about patients' biographies in an unprejudiced and thorough fashion, from conception to the day they walk into the clinic. This means that it cannot derive solely from the patient but must be amplified by other informants who know the patient and from corroborative data found in records from school, work, military service, courtrooms, and the like. All this material then must be reflected in the diagnostic formulation that makes sense of a patient's condition and presenting problems.

Psychiatrists following this path of induction discerned—contrary to the Freudian bias—that similar symptoms of mental distress could have very different derivations—some from brain disease, some from life encounters, some from vulnerabilities of personality structure, and some from behavioral habits, to name a few. Recognizing the various sources of distress and thus various therapeutic possibilities, psychiatrists could search across a broad range of information specific to each patient and enter into discussions and debates about diagnoses and assumptions in exactly the same way as do other medical specialists.

Subsequent to my education in neurology and psychiatry—and my immunization against sweeping explanations of mental disorder—my career path led me into positions where I was responsible for the education of others and the direction of psychiatric programs. At first I had to prove that my approach improved on what had come before under psychoanalysts. This proved relatively easy, especially as the discovery of medications such as lithium and antidepressants provided effective demonstrations. Along the way I fought other fads—such as when I was chairman at the University of Oregon Department of Psychiatry in 1973 and had to face down enthusiasm for "encounter group" therapy that was poisoning the interactions among the staff, patients, and resident physicians.

Essentially, as our accomplishments increased and people in authority saw that psychoanalytically inspired psychiatry was failing to unite practice and research (as Drs. Thorn and Adams had predicted), my students and I were offered progressively larger stages on which to work. I advanced from directorship to directorship in American academic psychiatry until by 1975 I was appointed the director of the Department of Psychiatry at the Johns Hopkins School of Medicine and psychiatrist-in-chief of the Johns Hopkins Hospital. We had at least persuaded the leaders of this distinguished university that our inductive approach could provide the compass the field needed.

By the mid-1980s, progress in psychopharmacology, genetics, and neurobiology had introduced other sources of information useful for making sense of mental disorders. However, the Freudian analysts had nested themselves within the broad framework of the discipline, usually by emphasizing that they offered a "humanistic" approach to patients. They did not give up their fundamental concepts, but they did not emphasize them as they interacted with students and residents and offered suggestions about patient care that had a ring of profundity.

Examples of this kind of camouflage include the following quotes from a Boston academic psychoanalyst, Elvin Semrad, who gained some fame as a pseudo-guru: "Don't get set on curing her, but on understanding her. If you understand, and she understands what you understand, then cure will follow naturally"; or "Find out what the heart says and where in the body the feelings are"; or—my favorite—"We're just big messes trying to help bigger messes, and the only reason we can do it is that we've been through it before and survived."

In this way psychoanalysts had settled into a comfortable if not very productive role in the psychiatric discipline. They continued to attract some disciples into their ranks, but no longer the more promising students. And many of them turned their attention away from the clinic and to the literature and humanities departments of the local colleges, where their ideas and interpretations were judged by what "illuminated" some text or fictional character and not by the objective assessing of premises or the testing of therapeutic claims by clinical results.

I was satisfied with this state of affairs, and thus, some years after I had settled into my position at Hopkins, I was surprised by the "recovered memory" idea that was to rip tragically and malevolently at the social and emotional fabric of many American families. For me it indicated psychiatry's sudden and unexpected reversion to the deductive explanations of mental disorders that I had by that time admittedly written off.

Again I was surprised—probably because I was too comfortable at Hopkins and assumed that the inductive stance had won everywhere—at the weight this movement carried with influential psychiatric authorities such as department directors, educators, and journal editors, despite the absence of any empirical support for the premise on which the practice depended. Many proved dogged in its defense and insulting to its critics (as my old teachers predicted). The whole affair demonstrated how vulnerable psychiatry remains to faddish practices and crazes—for reasons that I'll attempt to make clear as this book proceeds.

As I was to discover after the distressing experience with Richard Moore, the idea itself traveled under a variety of designations: "recovered memory therapy," "repressed memories of child abuse," "dissociative amnesia." Its champions taught that many adult patients consulting them for what seemed common forms of mental distress—depression, anxiety, marital disharmony, and the like—were actually and unsuspectingly suffering from psychological scars of cruel abuse they had endured at the hands of their trusted parents but had "forgotten." This childhood mistreatment, almost always sexual, had disappeared from the conscious memory of the patients because, said the enthusiasts for this new idea about the workings of the human mind, it was "repressed" into unconsciousness from the very instant it occurred only to evoke its havok in the form of the symptoms at hand.

Notice how these ideas represent a reversion to psychoanalytic themes (repression, the dynamic unconscious, symptom generation, and the like) but now clustered around a crude causal premise and, as I was discovering, a bizarre form of therapy. These therapists—copying the master Freud but lacking his genius—called to mind the 16th century Mannerist sculptors and painters who, imitating the earlier masters without their inspiration or skill, produced crude and grotesque works. I began to designate this misguided group as the Manneristic Freudians reckoning that the title worked to both describe their practice and indicate its derivation.

Like Freud, the champions of "repressed memory" (with its presumption of a flagrant, traumatic event or series of events in the patient's life history) did not develop their views inductively from witness testimony, follow-up studies, laboratory data, or any such compelling forms of corroboration. The idea was an axiomatic premise derived from the conviction that the symptoms of the patient—usually symptoms of anxiety, depression, or demoralization—could have no other source. Note the deductive syllogism: *premise:* symptoms of depression are products of sexual abuse; *observation:* the patient has symptoms of depression; *conclusion:* the patient had to have been sexually abused.

The therapists told the patients that successful recovery from their complaints of anxiety, depression, and so forth depended on the "recovery" or "recollection" of the memory of this abuse—an abuse that many patients not only failed to remember at first but even denied. "You must remember in order to heal," these therapists repeatedly told these patients. They took a probing, provocative approach toward the patients, often augmenting sessions with hypnosis and sedative medication to persuade them to abandon their "denials" and to dredge "memories" into consciousness.

As noted, these Manneristic Freudians repeated modes of classic psychoanalytic practice but differed in one crucial way. Here the therapists reversed the agency of disorder. Rather than the symptoms representing residues of the patient's *own* conflicted desires as an infant toward parents (those instinctive Oedipal feelings of sexual desire), these symptoms were the psychological expressions of the patients' victimization—the mental effects of the destruction of their trust and childlike innocence produced by parental betrayal and abuse.

With this change in the agents of mental disorders, the therapists created a monster they couldn't control. Their diagnostic deductions broke out into the public in a ferocious fashion that may have surprised some of them who had been accustomed to keeping their claims about patients and families restricted to the consulting room and the lecture hall, where they were not at risk. But given their proposal that many children had been subject to secret and vile tyrannies of the kind that would outrage anyone, they should have been ready for what transpired and shown more professional caution and prudence as they forged and promoted these opinions. Eventually the monster they created required them to move more and more into the public in support of their assumptions and thus expose their theory to scrutiny.

After all, crime revealed demands justice be done. And this principle soon evoked the criminal and civil systems of law, which, with much media attention, indicted fathers, mothers, and others and showered them with shame. It was too late for the therapists to retreat even if they had not intended to enter the kinds of public conflict that would ultimately reveal the inadequacies of their methods.

At the start, though, they transformed into an asset what on first blush seemed an incredible psychological opinion. "How could someone accuse her parents this way unless the accusations were true?" ran their argument. And yet the "evidence" consisted of vague feelings of "something happened," generated in a suspicious fashion, and devoid of any objective support, such as confirming witnesses, bodily scars, or records of childhood disruption.

All the elements of a persecution fell into place. Everyone agrees that child abuse is a vicious crime. Experts in a socially honored, caregiving profession were vigorously promoting an idea of unrecognized, widespread child abuse. This abuse, they said, now explained many hitherto mysterious, severe, and persistent mental disabilities. And, given that repression kept memories of abuse buried, many more victims need to be rescued and many other criminals, disguised as respectable men and women, exposed. Whether intended or not, a professional campaign of terror had begun.

And ready or not, I was drawn by the very path I had followed into the battles that this campaign would generate and up against opposition that I never had expected.

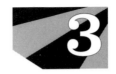

Appraising the Problem

I certainly sensed I was in a bad spot. I had been inattentive and stumbled into what boded to be a nasty fight. Just how nasty I would soon discover.

The onset, though, reminded me of the way commentators have described the unintended and unexpected genesis of the decisive Civil War battle of Gettysburg. A brigade of Confederate soldiers strolled down a small Pennsylvania road to commandeer shoes from the village. They bumped into a group of Union cavalrymen on patrol in the region. Generals Lee and Meade with their multitudes were miles away. But before they were fully aware of what was happening or how to maneuver, their forces were colliding and they had to scurry to unite their scattered armies for a fight that would turn into the biggest battle of the war.

Like those generals, when I first became aware of the emerging "recovered memory" faction, I wondered whether this was my fight. Maybe I should just let the Baltimore skirmishes settle, I thought. The movement appeared to have momentum, drew sympathetic backing by alleging overlooked and concealed child abuse, and would present a formidable challenge for any opponent to counter.

And yet it was such a terrible mistake. It would injure many families and damage public confidence in psychiatry. If I, the Psychiatrist-in-Chief of the Johns Hopkins Hospital, couldn't tackle this misdirection, who could—or might dare—try? The issue seemed clear: If not me, who? if not now, when?

But also like those brigade commanders, I needed help from an army. This was not a fight I could tackle alone as I had other, less sweeping psychiatric disputes over thought and practice. Those issues I had approached on my academic home ground, where I could draw up the agenda, organize the interactions, choose the case examples, and display success.

This issue would be fought outside of Hopkins; the skirmishes would spring up with little notice; and they would involve situations where my position and my administrative authority counted for little.

On the other hand, recovered memory therapy, although far more offensive in its suppositions than previously disputed treatments (and much more mean-spirited and destructive in its aims), grew in such a familiar way that I could easily say, "Here we go again." I had seen so many occasions where psychiatrists were encouraged to look into the "remembered" past of patients to find a buried cause of mental distress that I could anticipate the arguments these folks would put forward. I'd heard them before, knew how they would be woven into a specious logic, and appreciated their lure.

These were the arguments supporting the "unmasking" impulse of psychiatrists so strongly developed in Freudian psychoanalysis but hardly restricted to it. When psychiatrists take to "unmasking," they usually mention how they are not fooled by "appearances," how often "real" causes are overlooked, how mere fact-gathering is superficial, and how skilled one must become to discover sources of mental disorder "hidden from most" but known to them.

One of my favorite counterarguments to this way of assessing psychiatric patients, I took from an analogy Freud himself used in defending his practices. He would often picture himself as working like an archeologist, digging to find buried artifacts that would illuminate prehistory.

Indeed, I'd note, Freud was just like the early prehistorians who loved to attack an ancient site and drag out some treasure for all to admire. In the process they destroyed the site for future investigations and usually misconstrued the use and meaning even of the artifacts they tore from the ground.

Contemporary archeologists, I'd observe, carefully examine as they excavate, identify precisely the sedimentary strata they penetrate, and collect everything they find, right down to pollen grains. In this way they gather data and ultimately can illuminate the place, time, and purpose of every object—broken or whole, jewel-encrusted or plain—they find. They then can draw valid working theories about the sites they have explored and the stories these sites tell about prehistory.

The psychiatrists of today should be more like the contemporary archeologists—thorough, careful, ready to be corrected, quantitatively measuring what can be measured, low-key—and thus less like Freud. Those who, following Freud's example, "go after" something "big" in a life—be it sex, grief, trauma, neglect—will always succeed in pulling out something. But they often ignore how every life has sex, grief, trauma, and neglect in it. It's the context, specificity, and temporal relevance that provide salience to these matters and to all the other matters that form a life. What's "shoveled to the surface" may be—and usually is—incidental and ultimately trivial in explaining a patient's contemporary mental distress.

I'd had—and as I'll recount, still have—many occasions to draw on this archeological metaphor and cautionary tale. In a sense its lessons have been emblematic of my approach to teaching psychiatry.

I had come to Hopkins in 1975 by a path that encompassed clinical teaching and administrative responsibilities at other medical schools and hospitals—specifically in my roles as clinical director of the New York Hospital Westchester Division in White Plains, New York, in the late 1960s and early 1970s, followed by two years (1973–75) as chairman of the Department of Psychiatry at the University of Oregon Health Sciences Center in Portland, Oregon.

These were transitional years in American psychiatry generally. They included the discoveries of diagnostically specific, effective medications, such as antidepressants and lithium, and the growing need for psychiatrists to work with the most seriously ill patients to implement the "deinstitutionalization" policies launched by President Kennedy's Mental Health Act. It was my task to bring the implications of this transition to these centers—in other words, to return psychiatry to its medical roots in evaluations, treatments, and research.

My approach was always the same. I strove to alter the uncritical presumptions and practices of the department—usually some local ad hoc mixture of concepts vaguely tying together strands derived from Freudian, behavioral, and biological sources. I did this by generating an ongoing discourse over practice in which we would identify and criticize the methods of thought and procedure we were using.

I would try to teach everything anew, from the elementary—how to examine patients, corroborate the findings, record the results, and run the wards—to the complex—how to structure educational programs, design effective clinical rounds, and launch research programs tied to departmental interests. The aim here was to enhance the coherence, competence, and collegiality of departmental life always with a look to the future.

I encouraged everyone to abandon the idea that psychiatrists know a great deal. I thought we should realize that we were working in a rather rudimentary medical discipline, one that has few natural correctives, such as the autopsy room or the laboratory, to reveal its errors or restrain misguided enthusiasms. We should look closely at what we were claiming, in order that we might abandon what impedes and seize upon what advances our enterprises.

I didn't expel anyone from the conversations. I didn't stop anyone from presenting ideas, and in particular I didn't eliminate any theories, such as Freudian psychoanalysis or Skinnerian behaviorism, from being taught in these places. I just began to ask all practitioners to explain, with each patient they presented at rounds, the basis for their opinions so that everyone could decide whether that foundation was really as strong as was claimed or as appropriate to the matter at hand.

I was always happy to see successfully treated patients, but emphasized that I wanted to discern the actual source of success. I would be keen to note whether it rested on some tested idea of the practitioner that we could all learn to use, or whether the success came from his or her persuasive and kindly ways of dealing with a troubled person—ways that brought solace and help, but were hardly a specialist's monopoly or a new discovery.

I did, however, express my objection to certain habits of mind among practitioners. I let everyone know that I was not keen on expressions of the "unfettered imagination" when cases were discussed or causes proposed.

I would explain that imagination in psychiatric practice, where little can check it, is like violence in politics. It has an uncontrollable side, such that it thrives on the practices it evokes and transforms everything it touches into evidence to support its worth. Principles fade as imagination grows. Opportunists, cynics, and manipulators tend to prosper where imagination rules.

So I would tease my colleagues by saying, "I'm not immune to imagination; I have one of my own. But I like to keep it to myself and am allergic to its misuse—breaking into a psychic rash when exposed to imagination in the clinic."

In each of these places, within a few weeks of my arrival, the atmosphere and responses changed in such similar ways that they became recognizable to me, right down to the phrases chosen. Psychiatrists, it seems, tend to defend themselves with similar adages.

When I challenged a treatment plan, someone could be counted on to mention babies and bathwater. When I faulted a viewpoint, someone would invariably want to salute Werner Heisenberg and his uncertainty principle, which physicists use to explain their inability to measure simultaneously the velocity and position of subatomic particles. "Could we psychiatrists," he or she would ask, "not be entitled to similar leeway in our views?"

I would try to speak for the "babies" by encouraging practices of assessment that preserve what's important and real. And I, as patiently as possible, would point to the important difference between our studies with palpable human beings and those at the subatomic level, where the uncertainty principle rules.

But things usually heated up from there. People would demand to be recognized at a conference or round, only to announce how "tormented" they had become by the way the department was proceeding and how favorite programs were being challenged. "My friends are beginning to worry about my mental health and advise me to resign from this committee," one announced in the midst of a meeting to review the residency curriculum. He didn't resign, and his mental health seemed unharmed a year later.

Groups would barge into my office to explain why my methods troubled them. Their comments ranged from the New Yorkers' "You're taking my meal ticket away," to the Baltimorians' "Your close scrutiny of our practice is not in the Hopkins tradition of resident education."

On one occasion, when one of my faculty said that as a psychiatrist—and by that he meant one who "saw what others missed"—he had "no difficulty reading between the lines and discerning the purpose" of my proposals, I recommended the empirical approach by telling him to "read the lines and see if you understand *them.*"

Perhaps the most transparent way of resisting change that I heard repeatedly was, "It's not your ideas we are criticizing, it's your style." In this vein I had to listen—from liberal psychiatrists no less—to what amounted to slurs about how my ethnic origins made me naturally pugnacious and stubborn.

Most of the time, I saw these outbursts as ordinary responses to the implications of change, and I tried to reassure the protesters that their concerns were heard but were exaggerated, and then pressed on with my plans. I redirected everyone's attention to the most urgent issues at hand. Our department—and to some extent our discipline—was under notice that we must improve, and that required changing habits that were holding us back.

I was striving to change things, because change was required. The old ways were failing in the face of new demands on psychiatrists. At New York Hospital in White Plains, where I was given my first directorial appointment, the residency education program had been placed on probation, one step away from being discredited. At the University of Oregon Health Sciences Center and at Johns Hopkins, the psychiatric departments had failed both to provide excellent clinical services and to generate research. The departments were—not to put too fine a point on it—demonstrably incompetent.

But I intended to do more than simply make them competent. I planned to make them less doctrinaire and in that way more interesting. By ceding dominance to imagination and insubstantial theories, we had surrendered responsibility and overlooked the advances that were emerging from contemporary psychology, pharmacology, and neuroscience—programs of progress I pointed out that we ourselves someday might enrich.

I applied this stance with all the approaches to psychiatry—the psycho-dynamic, the behavioral, the pharmacologic, and the wishy-washy eclectic line ("use what you think works")—and at one department or another along my path I met them all. My main method was to use patient examples and ask for the approach to be applied to the specific case in front of us. "What do you know," I'd ask, "and on what basis do you claim to know it?"

I taught how a patient should be examined, a history taken, observations made, and factual claims corroborated from outside sources. I urged the use of quantitative measurement to strengthen our assessments. (We developed our own tool for measuring the cognitive state of patients that eventually came to be used by psychiatrists and neurologists throughout the world.[1]) I warned against drawing conclusions prematurely and encouraged explana-tions backed up by confirming, validating, publicly accessible information.

This brought the conversation down to earth—and in the process taught all who would listen the empirical practices I endorsed. And very shortly a series of successes in patient assessment and care—corrected diagnoses, more successful treatments, enlarged consultative power and scope—brought persuasive examples of the utility of this approach from the daily life in the hospital and the clinics.

Not everyone, though, was satisfied, and in each setting during the first year of my tenure some members of the faculty resigned and went elsewhere to teach. Some residents left the training program to seek other programs where, as one said to me, "there is less stress on what we don't know and more on what we do."

But things usually settled down within a year. Replacements came, saw that the expectations were not unreasonable, and discovered that despite how little we actually could claim in this discipline, the methods we taught worked well and had great promise. They saw that they now could—as all doctors must—identify what they knew, how they knew it, what it meant in practical terms of treatment and prevention, and how new research would most likely proceed. What seemed at first plodding enterprises of fact-gathering led to interesting, informed discussions that would evoke exciting themes from the realms of genetics, epidemiology, psychology, neurophysiology, neuroimaging, pharmacology, and the like.

Over time, as I had predicted, members of our group were drawn into these realms of study and ultimately became recognized as national leaders, adding new discoveries to them and deriving better practices from them. What had been obscure and difficult became more open and clear to us all.

Recruiting new associates is easy when you work in a flourishing academic medical center. Talented medical students flow through your services on assignment. If you can make your subject coherent and promising, they join you in growing numbers. Some are gifted clinical thinkers and stimulate the practice by sorting out difficult clinical problems. Others are more adventurous and begin research programs that illuminate for everyone some particular aspect of the work. All of them together can inspire enthusiasm for the work and add to the power of our enterprises.

And this is what happened. From each of the centers I led, I recruited young men and women and thereby built a small battalion of talent. We began growing at New York Hospital, then moved to Oregon and picked up others. When I was invited to come to Hopkins, I could bring along fifteen people who fitted various slots in the clinical, teaching, and research services and knew exactly what I wanted. They made the transition to Johns Hopkins smoother than the previous experiences. We were up and running more quickly because I had many others explaining the approach we were taking and why it worked.

———————◆———————

I recount these experiences as a prologue to my confrontations with the recovered memory movement because they both prepared me for it and revealed to me my awkward situation. I saw that this movement was a more baldly aggressive but similarly manipulative approach to that of the Freudians. The Manneristic Freudians strove to search the memory for past abuses rather than instinctive natural conflicts. Like the Freudians, however, they ran on a vivid imagination and generated amazing stories and claims.

But more pressing at the start was recognizing how much help I'd need in challenging this movement and just how isolated I was. From the very first incidents in 1990, I began to look around for allies and was surprised to discover that practices and ideas that I thought obviously amiss, few others seemed to see as troubling.

When I would point out the wildly improbable rise of cases of MPD (from the nineteenth century to 1982, only about two hundred had been found, but since then thousands have been, and all attributable to sexual abuse), many psychiatrists I spoke to would reply, "We're discovering new things I guess" or, "We're learning that anything is possible in a family."

I suggested that they were ignoring an alternative explanation: diagnosing MPD had simply become an intellectual fashion—one that would have tragic consequences for thousands of families and bring discredit to our profession. They would respond to this by noting that I might be right but, if wrong, I would be seen as supporting child abusers. Not a good reputation for a psychiatrist, they warned, and not one they'd risk themselves or advise for me.

A most telling example of my isolation was an occasion when I brought up my concerns about the unfolding recovered memory hysteria with another hospital director, only to have him reply: "You just don't understand dissociation." This pulled me up short. Although I'm accustomed to being told I'm wrong about something, I'm not usually told I don't "understand" a term common enough in psychiatric parlance.

What I realized is that I didn't understand dissociation in the way he did. I had seen it used by psychiatrists—and still do—in relation to patients who claim such things as having "amnesia" or having suffered from "fugue" states in which they wander from home and turn up miles away unable to explain how they got there.

If, when asked to explain the behavior of one of these patients, a psychiatrist says, "The patient dissociated," the word *dissociated* is merely a description with a professional ring masquerading as an explanation. One really knows no more about a case of amnesia or fugue by saying the patient "dissociates" than by saying the patient behaved as though he or she couldn't remember.

My friend was right. I didn't understand dissociation as he and the champions of MPD did. I thought it was a duplicitous term begging the question of why a recollection of trauma or abuse was absent in a patient where such abuse was presumed.

Mountains of evidence had demonstrated that shocking and frightening traumatic experiences are difficult to forget rather than difficult to remember. Holocaust survivors were the cases most of us had seen. Many of them would *prefer* to forget their mistreatment, but the memories of their vicious experiences remain and trouble their adjustment to the future.

Also, a clinician with any biological sense should wonder how natural selection could lead to psychological responses in which humans lose from consciousness memories of injuries and threat. It would seem counter to survival. Only that "unfettered imagination" I warned against could dream up a scenario where such loss of memory was advantageous.

But we psychiatrists didn't need to rest upon our clinical experiences and common sense. Excellent psychological scientists have investigated these matters by studying the cases of individuals who, having witnessed violent crimes, been terrified by gunfire, or wounded in assaults, were followed up months and years later. In the follow-ups, their memories of the events were detailed and accurate. Children similarly, if over the age of five and thus no longer in the period of infantile amnesia, retain memories of distressing, painful, and frightening events for years with striking accuracy.[2]

Thus I could see that the concepts supporting the recovered memory movement were uninformed and that much of the psychiatric tolerance being shown to it rested on sympathy for the alleged child victims and not upon any evidence of its validity. Even more, I realized that I would need to find some like-minded people if I hoped to be effective in confronting this set of ideas and practices.

Just as this last realization became paramount, I discovered allies in a newly established foundation in Philadelphia. This organization proved to be just what I needed, a godsend.

Dr. Martin Orne, who had supported my use of polygraphs with Richard Moore, was working from his position in the University of Pennsylvania with a Philadelphia-based group of accused parents. He conceived an association (ultimately named the False Memory Syndrome Foundation) that eventually was to do more than any other group to challenge and reveal the scientific, logical, and practical errors tied up in recovered memories and MPD.

Orne had impeccable credentials to spearhead a group of this sort. He also had the vision to see exactly what its mission should be, given what was needed at the time—a need I felt so intently.

As both a psychiatrist and a psychologist, Orne had investigated hypnosis and the phenomena of psychological influence over a forty-year career. When still an undergraduate at Harvard College in the early 1950s, he had shown what did—and did not—happen when a person, in the hands of a skilled practitioner, was lulled into a trancelike state by a hypnotist.

For example, he demonstrated that hypnotized subjects who were age-regressed (told under hypnosis that they were a child of, say, age eight or nine) didn't genuinely revisit or "live mentally" in their childhood years. These years were not—as some hypnotherapists presumed—indelibly fixed in their mind as latent memories that could be reawakened or "rejoined" with the help of hypnosis. Rather, when questioned by the hypnotist about what they saw in their "trance," the subjects reported childhood scenes synthesized from pieces of memory and facts of their life but constructed by their adult imagination and assumptions. They simply "made up" a picture of themselves at a given age to satisfy the expectations of the hypnotist and the hypnotic setting.

In later forensic work, Orne showed how hypnosis could encourage witnesses to "remember" events that were impossible for them to have seen or experienced. He explained that hypnosis increases a subject's suggestibility and so gives people undue confidence in the "memories" that are suggested to them while hypnotized.

Orne had played a definitive role in establishing the inadmissibility in court of recollections obtained during hypnosis. His research provided the foundation for a 1985 American Medical Association Council on Scientific Affairs report that described hypnotically-generated memories as less reliable than normal recall, and branded them unfit for inclusion in the legal process.

Orne always maintained (and provided many examples to prove his point) that any recollection retrieved under hypnosis required independent, empirical, public corroboration separate from the hypnotic sessions if it was to be relied upon. His experience-based counsel was regularly ignored by the psychotherapists employing hypnosis to "recover" memories of early life abuse in their patients.

When families in Philadelphia who had been accused of sexual abuse by their offspring—often through hypnotically induced recollections—approached Orne for advice, he recommended that they do more than build a support group. Since many were professionals in their own right—academics, lawyers, and executives—they could draw together to investigate the practices that had led to their progeny's wild accusations. Together they might come to study the scientific and clinical grounds on which the practices were built, judge the recovered memories from their foundations and their history, and draw public attention to the dangers inherent in these supposed "therapies."

Orne also believed that the families together—all of whom had had a common and distressing encounter with a misdirection of psychological thought and practice—could appeal to some of the best scientists and investigators whose work he knew was being published on hypnosis and suggestibility, memory science and clinical practice, truth and error in psychiatry. These researchers might accede to a request from the False Memory Syndrome Foundation (FMSF) to come together with the families as experts from the various fields they represented.

In this way the experts could learn from one another and see firsthand how, through ignorance, a serious form of psychiatric malpractice had been launched. By getting to know the people most affected by this malpractice, the experts would be inspired to challenge and correct it. And by encountering the experts and their research, the accused would recognize just how therapists had gone wrong and what they could do about it.

And that's exactly what happened. The foundation sprang into life and brought all the strengths of many talented people together. Distressed people found support and encouragement. Its advisory board came to be made up of nationally renowned scientific investigators, including psychiatrists and psychologists, who were ready to confront this misdirection of practice and thought in their essays, their books, their experimental studies, their academic interactions, and, ultimately, the courts.

Certainly that's what I saw when I first attended a meeting of the FMSF. I was introduced to scores of people who had been charged by offspring and by the professional leaders of the recovered memory campaign of having been—and let's be clear about what was at stake—incestuous pedophiles. Some were in imminent danger of imprisonment and financial ruin. All were threatened, mortified, and should have been terrified. (And I had thought I was the one who needed help.) But they had found through the foundation that they were not alone in this situation and that they were not powerless to fight this misdirection of psychiatric practice.

The FMSF was essential for me. I had found an army to join, an army with many vigorous combatants in its ranks. We were to work effectively and collaboratively in what one of our number (Frederick Crews, the distinguished English professor from the University of California) came to call "the memory wars."

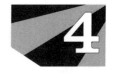

Joining the
Contest

In joining this enterprise I wanted to identify how my role as a clinician would relate to but differ from the efforts of the investigative scientists in the battle against the recovered memory faction. The scientists would—as I'll soon describe—reveal the shabby foundations of the ideas tied to repressed memories and their recovery. They would quickly devastate the notions as having little validity.

But that alone would not be enough, given that right from its beginnings Freud-inspired psychotherapy did not depend on scientific support and easily survives scientific criticism. Only challenges directed at the clinical practices (and the assumptions supporting those practices) would stop them and perhaps begin to teach the public at long last how to relate to psychiatry. This would be my role. A pair of contrasting clinical scenarios indicates why it was needed.

When surgeons tell patients complaining of abdominal pain that they should submit to having their appendix cut from their bellies, most patients, before they acquiesce, want to know the alternatives, the laboratory evidence backing the recommendation, and even whether a second opinion endorses the proposal. This scenario happens regularly, even though what is to be removed is a small, worm-like appendage to the gut, vestigial in nature and of little or no consequence. Only the cosmetic effect of the small, fading scar on the abdomen provokes lament.

But when psychotherapists tell patients complaining of depression or anxiety that they should submit to having their cherished and trusted fathers cut from their lives, nothing similar ensues, despite the enormous repercussions this proposal will have for their future. It seems that few demand a second opinion, ask for evidence, consider alternative treatments, or walk away. In one way or another, most patients go along with the plan.

At the level of everyday life, this second scenario, not to put too fine a point on it, is insane. But it actually doesn't occur at the level of everyday life. It transpires in the assumptive world that Peter Kramer identifies in his splendid short biography of Freud as the "modern mind" and that W. H. Auden called a "climate of opinion."

Three interrelated notions of Freud fed the "climate" early on and in one form or another still find approval among the culturally informed today. Freud taught and modernists believe that (1) mental distress derives from some hidden struggle over an aspect of sexual life, (2) the symptoms of distress symbolically represent that sexual problem or experience, and (3) the severity of the symptoms is directly proportional to the gravity of the difficulty.

 That none of these notions is true and all three were built on false pretenses (as many careful students of Freud have revealed) is beside the point here. They have had a lasting cultural effect on the public that extends beyond their particular claims.

They produced a persisting assumption that psychotherapists can be trusted in large part because they know deep secrets. Psychotherapy came to be seen as a universal balm that in a mysterious way would better us by calling from memory some inner ghosts and demons and exorcising them. The sources of these demons could be left to the therapists to discern.

This persisting assumption provided the easy perch for the Manneristic Freudians and their recovered memories psychotherapy. They could claim that they knew even more than Freud, saw deeper into the sources of inner demons, but in general accepted his three notions. At the same time, they could specify that sexual abuse of children by trusted adults caused the mental disorders and the symptoms displayed and that their severity was just what might be expected when one reflects on the meaning of sexual abuse to a child.

It was all so ready-made. When facing other authorities, such as the American Psychiatric Association (APA), these Mannerists could, like Freud, claim that their conclusions were drawn from what patients told them, that they merely continued emphasizing the centrality of sexual events in early life, and that, like him, they bore no responsibility for checking facts. Put this together with the modern mind's familiarity and trust in psychotherapy and the Mannerists had clear sailing both in official circles and with the public.

Pamela Freyd, the executive director of the False Memory Syndrome Foundation (FMSF), recalls that at first she and other accused parents assumed that the APA would denounce the recovered memory practices. "Why would they let it continue without saying anything?" she wondered. Hers was a natural enough expectation, but she didn't appreciate what she and all of us would soon be battling: the complex social and cultural presumptions present in American psychiatry and derived from the legacy of Sigmund Freud. They exist beyond the reach of science and more in the realm of legend.

I, however, thought the time was ripe to challenge the presumptions, transform the "climate," and rescue the "modern mind" from the folly of the repressed memory movement. These were initiatives that I, as an experienced clinician, could bring to the effort.

———————— • ————————

The launching of the FMSF in March 1992 was the first serious, publicly sustained, and methodical rejoinder to the recovered memory faction and its misdirection of psychiatric thought and practice. The foundation began by publishing a monthly newsletter updating the membership on scientific studies of memory and the course of the clinical battles. Its officers attempted to counsel accused parents via an 800 number about how to manage their emerging family crises. They directed confused and frightened people to thoughtful practitioners and to apt legal services. Most crucially, the foundation provided knowledgeable people drawn from its officers and advisory board to respond with letters and op-ed pieces for newspapers and magazines when reports appeared that presented one-sided child abuse stories based on recovered memories.

We all discovered that the mainstream media—long accustomed to accepting psychiatric opinions without challenge—was remarkably trusting of claims, especially from celebrities, of long-forgotten sexual abuse uncovered in therapy. *People* magazine ran a cover story in October 1991 about Roseanne Barr: "I Am an Incest Survivor," the headline read. Barr was following along the publicity trail of a former Miss America, Marilyn Van Derbur Atler, who also described recovering memories of her alleged abuse to the magazine earlier the same year. Oprah Winfrey devoted several sessions of her popular and influential show to "victims" telling their stories. She never asked whether people ever get the facts wrong when trying to recall memories in therapy.

As the FMSF offered rebuttals to these stories and the psychiatric opinions on which they rested, it drew critical attention to its efforts. The critics usually maintained that the FMSF was some kind of public relations front for sexual predators or that it was "clearly part of the growing backlash against feminism," as Cathy Wasserman wrote in an issue of *Sojourner* in 1992. But despite these insulting challenges, the FMSF grew rapidly.

A handful of families from Pennsylvania were in at the beginning and drew attention to the foundation. But the news spread, and membership doubled every two months, so that by 1993 over 2,000 people had called or written, eager to contribute to the effort, and almost every state in the country had a branch of the foundation. It obviously met a need for a forum where experiences could be shared and where information could be transmitted about the strange practices and claims of "recovered memories."

The new members wrote heart-wrenching stories of family relationships sundered after grown offspring, mostly female (90 percent of accusers are women),[1] "discovered" in therapy that they had been abused by their parents. These grown children began campaigns to hurt their parents using such cruel means as denying them opportunities to see their grandchildren, splitting off siblings, and hiring lawyers to demand funds for living expenses and psychotherapy.

The news of the FMSF spread to the media and was heard. Although many reporters reviled the foundation and many feminists attacked it because they believed "recovered memories" confirmed their views about patriarchal oppression in family life, three women (staunch feminists in most other matters) wrote compelling pieces about this misdirection of psychotherapy. They, true heroines firing the first salvos in the first battles, were Dorothy Rabinowitz, in *Harper's* magazine and the *Wall Street Journal*; Stephanie Salter, in the *San Francisco Examiner*; and Carol Tavris, a distinguished social psychologist, in the *New York Times*.

Each of them, on the basis of independent study, wrote compellingly and persuasively about how incoherent the recovered memory movement was in both theory and practice and about what serious damage it was doing. All three of these women had to overcome backlash from friends and fellow workers when they wrote their pieces. They were going against the stream, but did so bravely and effectively.

With their help, the term "false memory syndrome," coined by Peter Freyd, joined the parlance of the media. Official psychiatry (APA), although in the process of revising its *Diagnostic and Statistical Manual (DSM)* in 1993, held out against accepting the term. The pertinent *DSM* committee was headed by believers in buried abuse memories, and at the time they were concentrating on changing the diagnostic term for the mental disorder they believed was produced by those "memories" from "multiple personality disorder" to "dissociative identity disorder" (DID). They thought that by putting the concept of dissociation into the title they would identify what was being overcome when memories were "recovered." They would not countenance an official diagnosis for the false memory syndrome, as it represented a clear challenge to their assumptions about what exists.

The FMSF, though, had important things to do. Given the charge and vision of Martin Orne, it did not restrict itself to bringing public attention to the issue of false memories. It planned and vigorously pursued a mission of promoting scientific study and analysis that would enhance the understanding of how memory works and how clinicians' ignorance about memory played a role in these psychiatric mistakes.

The foundation took its first big step in fulfilling this mission by calling together as many experts as would agree to participate in a national conference on repressed and recovered memory at Valley Forge, Pennsylvania, in April 1993—essentially one year after the FMSF came into existence. The symbolic resonance of locating the first meeting where in the winter of 1777–78, during the American Revolutionary War, George Washington had encamped the ragged and struggling Continental Army did not escape our sense of the situation.

Like Washington's little army, the FMSF was also under siege. The organizers believed that gathering a group of interested people together would strengthen resolve even as it tested commitments. It would also indicate whether the FMSF was ready to burst forth as a coordinated, integrated group with sufficient authority to challenge the MPD craze.

Although only a small assemblage was expected by the original planners, the meeting's attendance topped six hundred. What a meeting it was. The discussants were not limited to those who objected to recovered memory therapy, but included several of its champions. Scores of scientists and clinicians presented their views and experiences. Hundreds of family members circulated, listened, and questioned them all.

I attended and met dozens of gifted people, experts in memory and social science, best-selling authors, civil rights lawyers, and concerned law officers, along with feisty accused fathers and mothers ready to reveal what they knew. All these people drew me into deep discussions—mostly on the methods of assessment behind my clinical opinions and what it would take to corroborate or challenge them.

They asked for my references, they wondered about my claims, they challenged my interpretations, and I loved every minute. This was the kind of interaction I had sought from the start—people responsibly looking for the truth and wary of losing sight of that goal because of their convictions. Two of these champions stood out for me that day and would later enhance my grasp of research surrounding psychiatry.

Dr. Richard Ofshe, a distinguished sociologist from the University of California at Berkeley, concentrates on social psychology and in particular on the way people can fall under the influence of others. During the 1970s he worked on the cults that emerged in that era, striving to understand how they succeeded in exerting their mind-altering influences on individuals.

Ofshe also examined police interrogation techniques. He was prompted to these studies by evidence—acknowledged by police and public critics alike—that these interrogations have on too many occasions provoked false confessions and distressing miscarriages of justice.

Of most pertinence to the FMSF conference was the decisive role Ofshe played in the case of Paul Ingram. Ingram, a respected sheriff's deputy in Olympia, Washington, had been charged with and, during intense interviews that included psychological suggestions, had come to "remember" sexually and physically abusing his children during supposed satanic cult rituals.

Ofshe was initially brought in by the prosecution because his knowledge about cults might help track this alleged satanic group. But when he examined the charging materials, the children's accusatory depositions, and the methods of interrogating Ingram, Ofshe transferred to the defense. He was convinced that Ingram, under intense police questioning, had become persuaded that he must be a person who "repressed" memories of sexual transgressions and that he should "try to remember" them. Although he struggled against this strange idea, he ultimately gave in to it and pled guilty to crimes against his children.

Richard Ofshe is a formidable man—the epitome of a stand-up guy. He conceived, essentially under fire from prosecutors who first brought him into the case, a way to reveal Ingram's vulnerabilities to suggestion and false memories. He invented another story of Ingram abusing his children and then, using the same methods as the previous investigators, succeeded in getting Ingram to accept it as true.

He essentially inserted false memories of his own devising into Ingram's memory. When he confronted the sheriff, police, and other law officers with all his evidence, he convinced them that a grievous mistake had been made. There had been no sexual abuse in Ingram's family, and no satanic cult in Olympia.

Ingram eventually recanted his confession, but his guilty plea could not be withdrawn. He served more than a decade in prison. The story of Richard Ofshe and Paul Ingram is well recounted by Lawrence Wright (a visitor to the Valley Forge meeting) in his book *Remembering Satan* (1994).

Dr. Elizabeth Loftus is another stalwart and gifted scientist I met at the Valley Forge meeting. She was at that time a professor of psychology at the University of Washington but today holds the title of Distinguished Professor at the University of California at Irvine. She has received many honors and achievements, including election to the National Academy of Sciences and the William James Fellow Award of the American Psychological Society.

Loftus began her career as a cognitive psychologist studying memory and memory distortion in the early 1970s, long before the recovered memory craze. Ultimately her work and what it revealed proved essential to the false memory battles—battles over ideas that had never even been imagined when she began in research.

Loftus has shown that even eyewitnesses can be unreliable when later called to testify to events. She demonstrated that the memory for a prior event can be markedly altered by giving witnesses incorrect information in the process of questioning them.

As she revealed how malleable and fragile human memories were, Loftus realized that the techniques used by psychotherapists of any school who encourage people to try to remember events from the past could easily create false memories. In what every psychology student knows as the "Lost in the Shopping Mall" experiment,[2] she demonstrated that some children and teenagers could be led to believe—by encouraging them to try to remember a story they thought came from their family—that when they were age five or six they had been lost in a shopping mall, had become very upset, but were ultimately rescued by passersby and reunited with their parents. Actually nothing of the kind had ever occurred. And not only was it possible to plant this false memory in about 25 percent of these subjects, but many of them embellished the story with extra details on its "recall."

Beth Loftus's achievements demonstrate how basic scientific research done primarily for its intrinsic value should always have, as hers did, public support. Without her work and the information about memory it provided, the FMSF would have had a weaker case to prosecute and a less effective model for demonstrating how faulty memories develop.

Her compelling findings strengthened the commonsense insistence that objective proof must back up and corroborate any memory of a past event. But her results and her conclusions were ill received by the champions of recovered memory therapy. They have striven ever since to disparage her research and argue against its clinical significance. In this way they demonstrate how little they understand either the critical role of experiment in contemporary psychology or how to respond to its results.

I came to realize at the Valley Forge meeting that Loftus is one of this world's natural wonders. An engaging woman with a feel for life's joys, she emits that sense of intellectual security that comes from long study and responsible, interactive scrutiny of informative research. I found her to combine a gift for friendship with the traits of a superb teacher and investigator.

Ofshe and Loftus were a sample of the talented people I met at Valley Forge. I had been asked to speak at the meeting because in 1992 I had identified in *The American Scholar* the frequent misuse of the multiple personality disorder diagnosis by psychiatrists and its treacherous link to recovered memories.

The organizers of the meeting asked me to go over this ground. I was asked to demonstrate how the diagnostic practices of the Manneristic Freudians deviated from what traditionally represented standards of care and also how those standards had evolved from trials and errors in the history of psychiatry. The intention was to show how the recovered memory faction was repeating old mistakes and, as Ofshe would note, "making monsters" in the process.

I saw my presentation then as a challenge—I had to show some of America's leading social scientists, psychologists, and psychiatrists that I could pass muster as an FMSF recruit. I made it clear how I wished to help them—and the besieged people being falsely charged—drive this misdirected set of ideas from psychiatry. I hoped they would embrace me and see my place in the campaign.

I spoke first on multiple personality disorder, describing with references how standard psychiatric teaching had—until Cornelia Wilbur spoke up in 1973—held MPD to be a human behavioral display provoked by suggestions and sustained in large part by the attention that doctors tend to pay to it. This means that it is not a mental condition that derives "from nature," such as panic anxiety or major depression. It exists in the world as an artificial product of human devising—an artifact of a most special kind.

MPD is a behavioral posture. It emerges and develops during the therapeutic exchanges between distressed people (with any of several different kinds of mental disorders) and their psychotherapists. In their quest for relief, the patients learn that proffering this representation of themselves captures the attention of the therapists; and the therapists, believing this posture represents an expression of early injury, guide them in shaping the stance and elaborating its expressions.

Thus, I said, every MPD patient presents a complex problem in which an artificial display has to be confronted and pushed aside so as to reveal the actual mental disorder behind it. An analogy of the clinical problem could be taken from William Butler Yeats's lovely poem "Among School Children": "How can we know the dancer from the dance?"

In order to clarify this matter, I considered the two issues of MPD and the recovered memories separately. Both rested on powerful methods of suggestion and belief inductions, including hypnosis, and both were intertwined.

I began with how good evidence confirmed the view that MPD was a behavioral artifact induced in patients by the doctors they sought out for help. The surge in MPD cases in the 1980s could be tied to the emergence and propagation among psychotherapists of crudely suggestive techniques to evoke multiple personalities in patients.

Therapists were told to use hypnotic inductions, barbiturate sedation, and isolation of the patients from other influences. They repeated questions to patients implying that other personalities must exist, and then rewarded the patients as the "alters" appeared by telling them that this appearance indicated recovery was under way. The nursing and social work staff would join in persuading them to think of their emotional states as expressions of different "personalities" and to give them names, one after another.

In some of their efforts to gain the patient's surrender to these ideas, the psychiatrists sequestered them on ward units where all the other patients were under the same kind of influence and had already begun to behave as multiples. Gradually, patients observing their ward mates and how they were responding—some in the most bizarre fashions, such as imitating animals or crawling on the floor like infants—began to follow suit and provide the expected multiple personality behavior.

I explained how similar these techniques were to those used by Jean-Martin Charcot in the 1880s, when he was misled by patients and credulous hospital staff into promoting the concept of "hystero-epilepsy"—demonstrating the symptoms of epilepsy without having the disease—and how the behavior surged among the group. I reviewed just how, after Charcot's death, his student Joseph Babinski had sorted out the truth.

I went over the lessons learned from this classic experience, including how doctors now realize that mentally disturbed people can easily take up what their doctors believe—especially if told that these ideas will help them recover. When patients are brought and kept together in hospital units where everyone—doctors, staff, other patients—accepts the belief system, then the beliefs will infect the new arrivals, spread in the group, and become more and more accepted by all parties. Patients may even compete to display the most vivid symptoms for the doctors' continuing attention.

Only other doctors can put an end to this kind of psychic contagion. First, they must break up the pooling of patients displaying these symptoms—in other words, no more separate ward units devoted to their "study." If patients are not well enough to go home and seek help individually in outpatient offices, they must be dispersed through the hospital on units that are free of other patients with the same symptoms. The patients cannot be witnessing other patients displaying these symptoms if recovery is to be expected.

Everyone must cease examining the patients in ways that are attentive to and provocative of the MPD symptoms. A kind of time-out must be brought into play, just as with other behavioral problems. With an MPD outbreak, this means no more talking to "alter" personalities, giving them names, describing their characteristics, and charting their interactions. Every single exercise that implies that these behavioral artifacts are real must be jettisoned from the exchanges between the patients and staff.

Simultaneously with turning their attention away from these themes, the doctors should direct the attention of everyone to other matters of concern. They should begin systematic inquiry with the patients and their relatives about "here and now" issues—considering recent encounters, previous illnesses, family history, social supports, vulnerable temperaments, and habits when dealing with life challenges. The clinicians must bring the patients to understand how these matters are actually the salient ones for them and let them know that the doctors, nurses, and social workers have many ways of helping them think about their situations and of dealing with them.

When, as they naturally will at first, the patients continue asking about the MPD features or even displaying what had previously caught the attention of the doctors, the staff need neither reject these complaints nor indulge them. All the members of the team—doctors, nurses, social workers, and other therapists—should tell such patients that these are but "remnants" of past problems from which they are now recovering and that these will fade as rehabilitation proceeds. A united front within the staff—of apparent uninterest in these symptoms even as the staff attends to and tries to help what's real in the patients' lives—wins the day. Patients recover and very often do so within a few days of instituting this new regimen.

After I had laid out these matters of comprehending and dealing with the manifestations of multiple personality disorder, I turned to the claims that these manifestations were products of repressed memory of sexual abuse that "split the personality" into "dissociated" parts. The methods for "recovering" memories were essentially the same as those for "discovering" multiple personalities. Here I strove to describe how clinically and logically dubious the claims were.

First and foremost, the trauma was usually assumed and not confirmed. Ever since Cornelia Wilbur brought forth the case of Sybil, her followers have taught that patients should be informed that MPD symptoms indicate that they had been abused (most likely sexually) by someone in their early life, that the MPD symptoms symbolically represent the "breaking up" of psychic integrity by the unacceptable nature of the betrayal, and that now, guided by the doctors and nurses, patients would recover as they remembered their history of abuse and who it was that had so injured them. (Note once again how this set of ideas mirrors the old three Freudian notions—mental problems rest on sexual issues, the expressions of the mental difficulties symbolize that problem, and the severity of the symptoms depends on the gravity of the conflict.)

I drew attention to the illogical elements in this theory-driven practice. The most obvious one—and one that emerges repeatedly (as we'll see later with post-traumatic stress disorder) whenever psychiatrists commit to a single cause for mental symptoms—is a fallacy well known and described by Aristotle: "affirming the consequent." This error of reasoning works on the assumption that if a particular event (A) can cause or provoke a situation (B), then any time one sees B, one can presume that A must have preceded it.

The error lies in an unacknowledged and undemonstrated presumption that A and only A can produce B. Many other events (C, D, E, etc.), different and distinct from A, could perhaps produce B and, because of the fallacy in reasoning, be overlooked, discounted, or even remain unsought upon encountering B.

Thus, even if one accepted that a particular symptom could be provoked by sexual abuse, that symptom would not denote, or represent indubitable proof of, a past experience of abuse. Many other events and other mental disorders could produce similar symptoms. Only with a demonstration that A actually happened to this patient and that C, D, and E did not happen could an argument for A as the cause of B be supported.

With their monorail presumptions about sexual abuse lying at the root of the MPD presentations (that they also induced), the followers of Wilbur have continued to use hypnosis, sedatives, and suggestion to send the patients on a quest for the culprits, whom theory taught the doctors to "know" were out there.

This quest distressed and disturbed the patients immensely, more so than the MPD displays. They were being instructed to develop, and then invest with detail, suspicions about their nearest and dearest relatives. "Try to remember" was the order of the day, and it was a painful process to undergo.

All denials were rejected and all failures in the quest construed as "resistance." The patients could have no contact with those members of the family who might have been part of the "abuse." Likewise they were forbidden contact with any other persons—such as previous psychiatrists—who might challenge the new diagnosis and "sustain the resistance" to its implications.

The patients' daily lives and whole existence turned on this quest for memories. All their "alters" shared in the responsibility for it and, often in hypnotic trances, were "questioned" separately for their "information."

It was chaos, of course, and gradually the patients' dreams, feelings, thoughts, suspicions, and daily behaviors reflected this chaos. They remained unsettled until they identified someone in their past as an abuser.

When this milestone in "recovering" memories was reached, their quest was not at an end. They were then encouraged, as a way of fully understanding their anxieties, their depressions, their marital difficulties, to build up long narratives of just how the abuse was carried out, who had participated, and how the patients had responded—a "script" of the abuse scenes that was to include their physical and emotional reactions. Here the therapists were emphasizing to the patients that they would recognize how their mental symptoms carried symbolic links to these experiences—obvious ones being how sex abuse translated into problems with marital intimacy, but more recondite ones being food antipathies, such as a dislike of pickles (cylindrical shapes longer than wide, don't you know?).

These scripts became catalogues of many incredible events. One patient told me she remembered being sexually molested during her bath as an infant younger than two years of age. She described her memory of being an enraged victim of a vicious rape who, because she was not yet able to talk, was "locked in" with her suffering and unable to call for help. Scripts of this sort were common and came to include rituals of group sexual abuse associated with devil worship, human sacrifice, blood drinking, and cannibalism.

I ended by describing how "flashbacks" and dreams were certainly not reliable evidence of trauma—sexual or otherwise. These were reflections primarily of what was on the minds of the patient and were, as psychotherapists knew well, influenced by what patients were talking about in psychotherapy.

Even in cases of known trauma, such as experienced on the battlefield, psychiatrists have—given the studies of John MacCurdy, an American psychiatrist in World War I—related these visions to stress-induced emotions. In his classic study *War Neuroses* (1918), MacCurdy describes how the dreams and visions of combat veterans were often depictions of more disastrous and ferocious events than those the soldiers had actually gone through. The dreams represented "anticipatory" fearfulness rather than a replication of an actual experience.

For example, the soldier might dream he was buried underground by shell bursts or overwhelmed by the enemy's troops. These were images resting on fears of what could have happened and might happen in the future if the battle situation didn't change. MacCurdy understood them as natural and protective psychological mechanisms that in ordinary life would encourage people to avoid situations in which they had been frightened.

The same reasoning applied to the so-called flashback dreams during recovered memory treatments. Those subject to such experiences were told that the dreams "proved" the abuse happened. How else could such visions emerge?

But the dreams are not evidence of an experienced event. They are evidence of the fears (and preoccupations with victimization) evoked and fed by the daily sessions of group and individual psychotherapy during which they and their fellow patients were urged to relive and recount scenes of trauma and betrayal.

Finally, I pointed out that only the weapons of investigative psychologists could decisively end this "memory war." They would have to confront the recovered memory faction with the facts it was ignoring, such as how memories are built and retrieved, how circumstances mold beliefs, and how hypnosis can mislead.

But the terrain of the battles in these wars would be the offices, the wards, and the educational conferences of clinicians (I had not then foreseen the law courts), where practice takes place and is justified. Here my role, along with that of several other experienced clinicians coming to join the FMSF, would be pivotal.

Armed by both our clinical knowledge and what psychological science

could teach us, we would demonstrate how the recovered memory practices were faulty both in the diagnosis of MPD and in the fictions of
"memory recovery."

But I wanted to emphasize how we were involved in something more
than medical malpractice. The recovered memory movement represented a
form of social madness. To consider it only a medical error of poorly trained
clinicians would be to trivialize it and evade its implications—like ascribing
the Salem witch trials to a misunderstanding among country lawyers.

These practices did not grow out of sand, but from deep assumptive roots
within the culture that should not escape notice or avoid censure. We had
much to learn and much to teach.

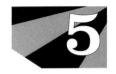

Fighting for Danny Smith

O ne early achievement of our work together was agreement on a definition of the false memory syndrome. This helped clarify the issue for everyone. The cognitive psychologist John Kihlstrom drew up the definition and passed it by us for approval. We believed it captured the matter well.

The definition asserts that the false memory syndrome is

> a condition in which a person's identity and interpersonal relationships are centered around a memory of traumatic experience which is objectively false but in which the person strongly *believes*. Note that the syndrome is not characterized by false memories as such. We all have memories that are inaccurate. Rather, the syndrome may be diagnosed when the memory is so deeply ingrained that it *orients* the individual's entire personality and lifestyle, in turn disrupting all sorts of

> other adaptive behavior. ... False Memory Syndrome is especially destructive because the person assiduously *avoids confrontation with any evidence* that might challenge the memory. Thus it takes on a life of its own, encapsulated and *resistant* to correction. The person may become so focused on memory that he or she may be effectively *distracted* from coping with the real problems in his or her life. (Italics mine)

This definition helped our cause escape indefiniteness by distinguishing among false memories and describing the attitude that patients with false memory syndrome develop and reveal. The words I italicized—"believes," "orients," "avoids ... evidence," "resistant," "distracted"—emphasize how patients' willpower and life direction succumb to the false presumption.

The definition spells out, as precisely as possible, the behavior of patients afflicted with false memories, but what it could not even begin to capture is that aspect of these patients that would ultimately drive our battles out of the clinics and into the courtrooms. It does not convey just how compellingly plausible these patients are when they present themselves as victims to others.

The aroused and agitated way they recount their stories would prove most telling, as it would usually overwhelm ordinary doubt. These patients express such misery and are so unwavering that most people who meet them are sure that something dreadful must have happened to them.

To advance the concept of false memory syndrome with the public, all these matters needed to be clear. We surely had to define the condition, but we also needed to indicate how those in the throes of this condition are overwhelmed by powerful feelings that spill out in any meeting with them to disrupt judgment.

I certainly had experienced the powers of persuasion these patients could wield. On many occasions—occasions when I knew how the "memories" had been generated and had information that rendered them impossible—I was awed, daunted to the point of being driven to recheck the facts, by the patients I met and the way they presented themselves to me. Their pitiful representation of their "memories" struck home and made withholding assent difficult. They are just so passionate in their claims, so insistent on their validity, and so clamorous for support.

Here is how the situation appears to anyone assessing these patients. They are usually young women, they are always emotionally upset and tearful, and they want more than anything else for you to join with them in their assumptions. Often the first question they want answered, even before they tell their story, is whether you "believe" in such phenomena as MPD and repression. They maintain that only fellow believers in these concepts will understand what they are about to describe.

They certainly do not seem "crazy." Their perceptions are not deranged by hallucinations or their thinking by confusion or irrelevance. They are educated, their choice of words precise, and their etiquette and responses to the moment intact. In every way other than in their beliefs and the "memories" that generated them they seem normal.

But with these beliefs they are resolute, unyielding. They vary in how long they will tolerate any hesitation or reserve on the part of an examiner. Some, as mentioned, insist that you pass an "advocacy test" and will not sit for an interview without hearing some expression of belief in the matters at issue, namely the authenticity of MPD and its production by repression/dissociation.

Others will at first forgo such a stance if an examination is demanded by some aspect of their situation. It may have been forced by parents from whom they are asking financial support or by lawyers involved in their litigation. Occasionally they present themselves for examination because they want help with other symptoms, such as persisting depression or anorexia, that have not improved despite their "successful retrieval of the memories."

But soon into any critical examination—even one begun with every effort at reassurance—all of them become restless and clamor to know whether they are winning endorsement. One brought a recorder to transcribe my responses to her questions because she wanted to be able to record what I said at the start of the interview that she considered supportive so she could play my remarks back to me if subsequently I wavered.

All kinds of emotional expressions, verbal and nonverbal, pour out of them—tears, shouts of anger, grimaces—all aimed at winning endorsement. These are followed—if their hopes for backing are unrequited—by cold disdain, condescension, derisive comments on the examiner's intellectual capacities and professional credentials. They repeat how they are victims of a cruel and vicious mistreatment and demand to know how you can listen to them and question anything.

Eventually it dawns on you that the meeting differs from customary psychiatric consultations in being a conflict of wills, and not a subtle one. Rather than allowing you, the physician, to sort out and settle on a diagnostic opinion, it has become an exercise intended to force or seduce you into validating a particular verdict. Only the most strong-minded and experienced of examiners can resist this pressure for affirmation.

What's at stake is a whole set of beliefs and opinions that the patients subscribe to and want confirmed. They resent being questioned about inconsistencies. If reassured at the start, they are quick to notice any wavering of that support.

They explain away any evidence of their past affection and gratitude for the parents they are now vilifying—expressions found in letters, cards, diaries, and the like—by referring to the "blindness of repression" at the time those expressions were made. They mention events that all can verify—such as household incidents that seemed innocent at the time, like domestic nudity, accidental bathroom intrusions, or jokes about sex—but give them significance in retrospect, holding them up as signs of the serious and secret abuses that they now recall through treatment.

They are quite simply fanatical about their opinions, and they insist that all their present difficulties in life derive from and are the effects of these "remembered" abuses. It is difficult for anyone (particularly for a doctor accustomed to consoling the injured) to avoid offering them some comfort. But imagine how difficult an effort to console can be, when striving not to agree instantly with their sense of the situation so as to ponder it.

It is pointless to argue with them, as doing so terminates the meeting. One does best by trying to fashion a link that encourages further engagement, such as by turning the patient's attention away from the memories and toward some particular symptom that might be helped by specific treatment.

Sometimes by working with depressive feelings or anxiety, one can draw these patients into care and gradually let doubts about their "memories" emerge either spontaneously or with careful countersuggestions.

This approach was employed with some success by my student and colleague Dr. Angela Guarda, who directs the Johns Hopkins Eating Disorders Program. Many young women with anorexia nervosa admitted to her care had been persuaded by previous therapists to interpret their anorexia as an expression of MPD and thus to assume that they had been victims of child abuse.

When these patients demanded that the treatment program explore those matters, Dr. Guarda would in one way or another respond by saying, "That's too tough for me. I think we should work on your eating disorder and how it has produced your starved, emaciated, weakened physical condition. We can return to these other worries after you've regained your strength."

Almost all her patients would accept this proposal—and, mirabile dictu, within a week or so the MPD and thoughts over abuse usually faded away. At least for these patients, the case is strong for concluding that their anorexia nervosa was not caused by "hidden sexual abuse." Rather, their susceptibility to the false memories came from their lowered resistance to suggestion when starved and depressed by anorexia nervosa.

Nonetheless, my experience with patients who related memories of abuse dispelled any surprise I once felt about why sympathetic listeners give in to these ideas about recovered memories. The patients, being convinced themselves, are convincing to those who work with them.

In later efforts to teach how people with "memories" can persuade kindly intended, sympathetic psychiatrists to believe the incredible, I pointed to the story of Dr. John Mack, a friend from my Harvard Medical School years. He ultimately became a professor of psychiatry at Harvard and achieved recognition both as a psychiatrist and as an author. (His biography of T. E. Lawrence won the Pulitzer Prize.)

And yet this gifted man was absolutely persuaded by patients who told him they had been abducted by space aliens and sexually abused on their spacecraft in the interplanetary regions. In fact, he was quoted in the October 11, 1992, issue of the *Boston Globe* as saying, "It's a question of clinical judgment. ... When memories come back like that I never have *any* question that these people are describing something that has *authentically* happened to them. ... No one has been able to come up with a counter-formulation that explains what's going on" (italics added).

When Mack was confronted by his Harvard Medical School superiors for evidence supporting such strange and wild clinical judgments, he was not at a loss. "Don't you believe in psychological evidence?" he replied, as though it was not the psychological "evidence" that was under question.

Eventually, Susan A. Clancy, an investigative psychologist at Harvard, looked into this matter in a searching and empirical fashion. As Dr. Mack should have done, she went beyond the testimony of the patients and any psychological presumptions to explore how their beliefs were evoked by considering the social contexts and characteristics of these patients, and the many life experiences they had suffered. She concluded and reported in her book, *Abducted: How People Come to Believe They Were Kidnapped by Aliens* (2005), that "alien-abduction memories are best understood as resulting from a blend of fantasy proneness, memory distortion, culturally available scripts, sleep hallucinations and scientific illiteracy aided and abetted by the suggestions of hypnotherapy."

Although I was reassured by Clancy demonstrating that a capacity for coherence still lived in parts of my alma mater, I regularly told the story of John Mack to emphasize how remarkably plausible patients with false memory syndrome can be and how this feature of them draws many intelligent people to their side.

But the story of Mack demonstrates only how beliefs in the impossible can occur. I was frequently reminded that most patients with false memory syndrome were remembering child sex abuse and not alien abduction and that child abuse was not an incredible claim.

Certainly sexual abuse of children does happen. Several reputable surveys of the population agreed that about 20 percent of women have had some form of unwanted sexual experience forced on them, especially during childhood and adolescence. And that such sexual abuse can have long-term adverse effects is established beyond doubt. And certainly we all agree that the persuasiveness of the victims does not undermine their claims.

In fact, this combination of the possibility of child abuse (and its pernicious nature) and the compelling appearance of the professed "victims" would determine the direction that the recovered memory conflict would take. It would also demand that all of us involved at the FMSF work hard to explain our point of view and make clear what we were and were not claiming.

In the battles over false memory syndrome, none of us was claiming that child abuse does not happen. We were claiming that accusations of child abuse derived from suggestive psychotherapy had to have more support than the plausibility of the therapists or the compelling stamp of the emotional displays.

A devastating experience, though, taught me—and many others—just how hard these distinctions were to make, and why many of our battles would eventually be fought in courtrooms and demand all of our expertise. It made two things very clear. First, I should never underestimate the power of conviction these patients project, and second, I should never overestimate the commitment of courts of law to rules of evidence. The event, like earlier ones, came without preamble.

I heard of the plight of Ray and Shirley Souza from Lowell, Massachusetts, one evening in January 1993. Their lawyer called me at home without warning to ask if I could testify for his clients. He described them as a married couple, retired and in their sixties, whose daughter had recently accused them of sexually abusing her as a child and had further charged that they were now abusing her and her brother's offspring, their grandchildren.

The daughter admitted that the memories of her abuse emerged in dreams during her psychotherapy. But then she said that, given her suspicions, she had questioned the children repeatedly and eventually gotten them to admit to ferocious experiences: of being kept naked in a cage in the grandparents' basement, of drinking green potion to make them sleepy, and then of being molested by a machine as big as a room.

It was bizarre and unbelievable. But I never met the accusers and thus could not judge exactly how they would come across in a courtroom. Never again!

I did not believe that a judge would countenance this prosecution without confirming evidence. I was busy with my duties at Hopkins and reassured the lawyer that he had little to worry about. He didn't need me to come up to Massachusetts. I told him that any trained psychiatrist would examine the accusing daughter and help the courts see the situation for what it was.

How foolish. The case came before a judge, Elizabeth Dolan. But after hearing the accusations and treating the defense expert witness Dr. Richard Gardner in a most hostile fashion when he pointed out inconsistencies in the testimony and the misuse of sexualized props such as anatomically correct dolls, she called for no objective evidence. She was certain that Ray and Shirley were two incestuous pedophiles, pronounced them guilty of the crimes, and sentenced them to house arrest.

I was thunderstruck and guilt-ridden. I had not foreseen how powerful a child abuse charge can be in a public courtroom and how, if not combated with vigor and expertise, it can undermine the good judgment of those assessing the situation.

By not challenging the validity of beliefs and demanding some concrete evidence other than the daughter's testimony, Judge Dolan was essentially putting the burden of proof on the accused. The Souzas in her view must demonstrate that they had *not* abused the children.

How were they to do that? The daughter presented no physical evidence of the crime, such as the cage, machine, or potion bottles. The purported victims displayed no broken bones, bruises, blood loss, or tissue injury. The Souzas were challenged to "prove the negative." They carried this practically impossible burden because the accuser presented herself in a most compelling fashion and because the accusations appeared to have psychotherapeutic authority behind them.

The Souza case made much clear. The only way to attack this misdirection of thought and similar miscarriages of justice was to attack that special standing carried by the psychotherapists. And, given the apparent acceptance of their ideas in psychiatric circles, the place for that confrontation would likely be in courtrooms.

Expert psychiatrists and psychologists had to come into court and testify against using recovered memories as an infallible foundation for any accusation. They must recommend that if such memories launched a charge, then they should be given no more special standing than other accusatory claims. To be credible, all such charges should be accompanied by solid, confirming, independent evidence of the claimed abuse.

Charges of sexual abuse must become, as I was to say many times, an empirical matter, with any confidence in their truth contingent on demonstrated facts. Recovered memories should cease being a matter of stories, anecdotes, and intense feelings.

In the climate at the time, achieving these aims would not be easy. And the reasons for the difficulties were of considerable interest in themselves, even though what they revealed was how we in the FMSF were on our own.

Official psychiatry was not ready to help. The editors of psychiatric journals and organizations such as the American Psychiatric Association were always uncomfortable with conflicts of opinion among psychiatrists. They worried about the discipline breaking up into warring camps and habitually opted, as they did here, for a political rather than empirical solution by presuming that truth over matters where clinicians disagree resides somewhere "in the middle" between the claims of partisans on the "extremes." (Harvard psychologist Richard McNally would later teasingly analogize this self-righteous and seemingly "balanced" posture as like striving to settle the controversy between those who believe the earth to be round and those who believe the earth to be flat by concluding that it's best to think of it as oblong.)

The culture itself was set up against us in a fashion that would influence judgments. The cultural viewpoints of insight that had given Freud purchase back in the 1940s and 1950s had been augmented since the revolutionary 1960s by attitudes carrying a more paranoid streak and that identified our society as built upon victims and antagonists of various sorts: victims of the patriarchy, victims of class war, victims of minority bias, victims of Western "hegemony." A psychotherapy that unearthed other victims had little difficulty finding support: it was telling a familiar story with a familiar assumption to a ready culture.

As for me, I would be entering an unfamiliar territory, one in which the settling of controversies ran on different conventions than those of the clinic or classroom. Judges and juries are not students eager to accept instruction, or ready to collaborate in developing the explanation of a problem. They were skeptics who'd probably rather be somewhere else, and who were committed to being evenhanded in assessing all the propositions before them—mine as well as the opposition's.

I would come to see just how much higher the stakes were in court than in my classes. After all, a poor round of teaching today can always be corrected by a better round tomorrow, but a less than stellar performance on the witness stand could send the people you came to help directly to jail.

Despite my misgivings about venturing into the courtroom, I came to perceive, as had other members of the FMSF, that we had to follow the cases into court, learning just what kind of public forum a courtroom represented and working for what benefits we could find.

The torment of the Souzas—and how I, in my naïveté and preoccupations, had left them to the mercies of an unmindful Massachusetts jurist—stirred my conscience and prodded me into courtroom work. There was nothing else to do but enter the fray and make the best of it.

The next opportunity came at me more directly, and I approached it, detail by detail, better prepared. One sunny Saturday afternoon in September 1993, I was sitting on my back porch in Baltimore when the doorbell rang. I found standing on the doorstep a middle-aged man who introduced himself as Danny Smith, the father of three teenagers. He lived with his family in Lexington Park, a small town in St. Mary's County in southern Maryland. Mr. Smith told me that in two weeks' time he would be going on trial for sexually abusing his daughter, Donna Smith, a nineteen-year-old who was currently a patient at Sheppard Pratt Hospital. He asked if I would speak with his lawyer, contribute to his defense, and perhaps save him from a long prison sentence.

"I don't know you, and how do you know me?" I asked. Mr. Smith had read a magazine article about my encounter at Hopkins with Dr. Loewenstein and how I wasn't a fan of recovered memory therapy. He had looked me up in the phone book and come to my house unannounced because he was desperate.

The woman who had been sitting in the car then approached me. She was his wife, Judee. "You have to understand, we're in despair," she said. "He could go to jail for twenty years. He's already lost his job, our other two children have been removed from our home, and all over claims that are not true but we can't fight."

It was a grim moment: this modest couple reduced to begging on a stranger's doorstep. I let them in to tell me more.

They explained that their daughter had had psychological problems throughout her adolescent years—depression, irritability, anorexia—but that it was only once she began seeing a therapist who believed in multiple personality disorder, and strongly suspected Donna suffered from it, that any suspicions had been cast on Mr. Smith. This therapist's contention had been reinforced after Donna was committed, by the State of Maryland, to Sheppard Pratt eighteen months earlier.

"What happened to Donna fits with what the magazine said was your opinion about MPD," commented Mrs. Smith, "that the doctors suggested this to her, that they wanted her to believe it."

After listening to them for a few more minutes, I promised to at least call Danny's lawyer in Lexington Park, Maryland, a Mr. Spaulding, to confirm their situation and what they were claiming.

During my call the following day, I learned many of the details about the Smith family situation from Mr. Spaulding, and these details ultimately were expanded when I reviewed the records submitted for the case. On the basis of those details, I decided that I would take the case, and this time I would be ready to confront both the misdirections in psychiatry it represented and the compelling characteristics of a patient with false memory syndrome.

The facts were these. When Donna was fourteen, in 1988, she was concerned about her frequent headaches and suspected that she might have bulimia. She was also depressed enough to ask her parents if she might seek psychiatric help. The family also noticed Donna was jealous of the attention that her younger brother with learning disabilities was getting from therapists and counselors.

In her search for help, Donna saw a number of different therapists over the next several years and was even hospitalized a few times. The diagnoses varied: on one occasion it was depression and bulimia—another time, anorexia and depression.

Despite these interruptions, she did well in school and enjoyed playing sports and volunteering for a local rescue squad. In 1990 her family physician recommended she see a new therapist, a mental health worker named Catherine Meyers, to cope with her eating disorders and her family relationships, especially her conflicts with her younger brother.

Ms. Meyers began early in her treatment sessions to ask Donna questions about whether her father had abused her. Donna reported later that Meyers had told her that women with eating disorders often had a history of being abused as children and that she wanted to look into this with Donna "just to check."

This line of questioning never found support from Donna until 1991, when Donna began to argue with her parents about how much freedom she could have, and what direction she should take in the future. She wanted to go to boarding school to get away from her parents' supervision—they ruled it out as beyond their means. These conflicts between the teenager and her parents provided some energy to the therapy visits that reawakened suspicions in the therapist, who began again to probe for sexual abuse.

In the summer of 1991, Meyers, with no new or transforming information or symptom presentation, changed Donna's primary diagnosis from bulimia to that now emerging popular diagnosis "post-traumatic stress disorder" (the history of which I will review in a later chapter). She told Donna that she believed someone had hurt her as a child but that, "as theories revealed," Donna might not remember it.

In their weekly sessions, Meyers continually asked Donna about the possibility of incestuous abuse from either her older brother or her father. She recommended that Donna read several books about surviving incest. And she asked Donna to bring in photo albums from her home so they could look at pictures of her as a child. (It's important to note that Meyers was not a doctor—neither a psychiatrist nor a psychologist—but rather a licensed mental health counselor.)

The albums proved the "trigger" that Meyers had been so doggedly seeking. When she and Donna were looking at the photos together, Meyers observed that Donna didn't look like a very happy child. At that point Donna said that maybe her father had touched her inappropriately once when she was little. When Meyers responded that she had to report this incident, Donna immediately recanted. "I'm lying, I'm lying," she said. Despite Donna's retraction, the therapist called the St. Mary's County Department of Social Services, and instructed Donna to remain in the office until someone official came. Donna ran out of the office and the building—but Meyers was able to catch her and hold her until the law enforcement agents arrived.

A social worker and a sheriff's deputy interviewed Donna that afternoon. When asked if her father had abused her, she replied, "I don't think so." The matter was dropped by the officials for a few days, but the family was not informed about the incident at Meyers's office or about how suspicious people had become about them as word of the incident spread in the Social Services Department.

Shortly thereafter, Donna and her father argued—on this occasion over that familiar adolescent issue, the use of the family car. Donna was agitated and upset the next day at school, and the guidance counselor had her call Meyers, who had her come to the social services office. There Meyers confronted Donna with what she had said before, noting that if she recanted the accusation against her father, people would never believe or trust her in the future.

All this led the social services to demand a court hearing, where it was decided to remove Donna from her home and place her under "protection."

Once out of her parents' house, Donna fell more and more under the influence of Meyers, speaking with her on the phone every day and going to her office for therapy three or four times a week. They discussed Donna's tendency to "dissociate"—Donna described it as living with a ghost floating above her—and about MPD and post-traumatic stress disorder.

Knowing about the interest in MPD at Sheppard Pratt, Meyers took Donna to the hospital for a consultation over the MPD diagnosis. In the interview in Baltimore, Donna behaved in ways depicted in the movie *Sybil*, which she had seen in her high school science class, and that Meyers indicated were typical of MPD patients. She would change her voice and move her position in her chair as she adopted different "alters."

Soon after this visit, the county officials decided to admit Donna to the hospital, where she could receive care and "protection" on the ward devoted to multiple personality cases.

As I would testify at the trial of Danny Smith, Meyers failed fundamentally in her care of Donna. A high-strung and volatile teenager who in the past had struggled with an eating disorder and depression is far more likely to be continuing to face those issues and to need help in her developmental struggles with her family than to be suffering from anything as exotic as MPD. Instead of recognizing and treating Donna's depression, Meyers introduced her to false ideas about her father and incest and then encouraged her to buy into those beliefs by promising her recovery.

That was the first—huge—error in Donna's treatment, but it was compounded by the doctors at the hospital who furthered these errors with a bizarre course of treatment for Donna. For a few days in the admission unit she saw doctors who were not ready to accept the diagnosis of MPD and were of a mind to meet with her parents to discuss the allegations of sexual abuse.

But for reasons still unknown—perhaps in part because of Donna's own demands when she turned eighteen a few days after the hospital admission—she was transferred to the hospital's MPD unit, where doctors more in agreement with Meyers refused all visits to Donna by her parents. The doctors also refused to check with others on Donna's reports of the facts and her past clinical history.

Donna began seeing the chief of the unit, Dr. Loewenstein himself. But not long into her treatment, she confessed to him that she was lying about her father's abuse of her and that she had lied about everything. Like Meyers before him, Loewenstein refused to accept her statement. He told Donna that if she was lying, she was much sicker than if she had MPD.

The personnel on the MPD unit reinforced the diagnosis in the typical way: helping Donna to "name" different actions or feelings so all her different "personalities" could be identified, hypnotizing her often, telling her that as she explored her psyche she would uncover more and more of the past—and that she would react with rage, sadness, and feelings of helplessness.

When indeed these feelings did emerge in the course of their treatment, the psychiatrists prescribed sedatives such as the benzodiazepine drug Klonopin. Because Donna was given very high doses of these sedatives, she was essentially "drunk" through much of her hospitalization.

The unit's doctors and nurses began to suggest not only that her father had abused her, but that perhaps her parents were members of a satanic cult, and that she had been subject to "satanic ritual abuse" as a child. This naturally caused her and others to worry about her brothers, who were still living at home.

From February 1992 until the following June, Donna never saw her family. None of the doctors on the unit thought it wise to check in with Donna's parents, or to let them come and see their daughter. Isolated, often drugged, and haunted by what she believed had been done to her as a defenseless child, Donna was frequently wrapped in wet, cold sheets for hours. This wet pack treatment—a throwback to nineteenth-century and early twentieth-century methods of restraining agitated patients—did subdue her outbursts.

In June, the consequences of Donna's therapy began spilling into the outside world. Someone at the hospital called the sheriff's office in St. Mary's County to report that Donna's brothers were in danger of satanic ritualistic abuse from their parents. Three deputies went to the Smiths' house and removed the boys—in handcuffs, since they would not leave willingly. Meanwhile, Danny Smith was charged with child abuse. Preparations for a trial began.

Danny's lawyer, when I first talked with him on the phone, was worried about the case. Although Mr. Spaulding believed his client innocent, he knew the hospital was planning to send down its leading doctors to testify for the prosecution. He'd been told they would testify that only severe parental abuse could have brought Donna to her current state, where wet pack treatment was "necessary."

He sent me what records he had so that I could review them and formulate my own position on Donna Smith's mental health and the diagnosis of MPD that had been made in her case. There I learned how her parents had taken Donna from therapist to therapist from age fourteen onward. Would they really have done this had they been abusing her? I also saw that no therapist before Meyers had ever suspected child abuse. Could so many previous therapists be wrong and only she right? It was possible, but unlikely given the claims of serious and continuing ritual abuse.

I also read with interest the diary that Donna kept, starting at age fourteen, which her parents gave to me. In one entry she wrote:

> Some people think I have everything going for me. Good grades, *not child abused*, nice things, parents spoil me to death, great plans for the future and much more, but they don't see the other side of me. The side of me that is hurting badly inside and longing for love and a real mother, who understands me. (Italics mine)

It was hard to miss the fact that she explicitly states she had not been abused, and that the focus of her discontent was her mother, not her father. I asked her mother to explain the background of this entry, and she recalled that she and her daughter were quarreling at that time, mostly over trivial matters, such as her responsibility for some of the household chores.

A later entry also caught my eye:

> I wish I had something to blame this on.

Donna, it appeared to me, was struggling with low feelings from her depression and with common teenage developmental issues, such as forging some independence and fighting for privileges.

Perhaps she didn't persist in rejecting Meyers's suggestions of sexual abuse because they provided "something to blame this on." Also, when in the midst of her depression, she was more vulnerable to accepting the idea of MPD. At least this way of thinking about her and her situation would make sense of the evidence shown to me.

But this evidence was not in front of the doctors at Sheppard Pratt. The Smiths told me that from the time Donna first went to the hospital, they attempted to reach the doctors and discuss her previous problems, their experience with her, and their family life in general. The Smiths particularly noted that they brought the revealing diary, along with other documents about Donna's history, but no one in the hospital—doctors, nurses, or social workers—would look at the documents or listen to what the parents had to say. They considered all these matters unimportant, given what Donna was saying and doing on the wards.

As I later testified, the doctors' disregard of the family reports meant that all their diagnostic opinions—traumatic sexual abuse, repressed memories, satanic ritual abuse, MPD—rested not on objective evidence but on speculative theories built around the displays of this distressed young woman—displays that they themselves had helped encourage.

The isolation they imposed on Donna also enhanced the powers of suggestion and indoctrination. This was reinforced by daily therapy and group discussions about MPD on the ward.

Cut off from other influences and surrounded by fellow patients who talked endlessly of their own supposed "alters" and abuse histories, Donna became totally convinced that she had MPD. Various exercises, like naming the alters as if they were real people, diagramming their interactions, and supposed linkages to each other and to the "abuse" memory on vast charts, even setting up bulletin boards where one alter could leave messages for another, (all standard practices on the unit) strengthened her beliefs in the "system of alters" that represented her MPD.

In addition, regular hypnosis and sedative dosing kept Donna in a state of mind that made it easy to convince her of the truth of her beliefs and sustained the idea that she was a victim of her parents' malevolent behavior.

The Smith trial took place in a brick country courthouse in Leonardtown, Maryland. After explaining to the court that she had chosen five personalities—"helping alters"—to use while testifying, Donna described on the witness stand the abuse she allegedly received at the hands of her father. Meyers and the hospital doctors also testified to the likelihood of the abuse and what Donna had told them about what she remembered when she was under their care.

Danny Smith took the stand to deny the charges. I came down several days into the trial, having read the testimony to that point. In a diner near the courthouse, I met with attorney Spaulding and we outlined on a paper napkin the points I wanted to make.

I told the court I believed Donna suffered from an induced hysterical disorder. Under the direction and the suggestive encouragement of her doctors and the other members of the ward staff, she had come to imitate the symptoms of someone with a mental illness and believe she suffered from it. Her counselors and physicians had taught Donna to act as she had and then in many ways had encouraged and sustained her in the behavior.

The capacity of humans to imagine and imitate illnesses has been known to doctors for centuries, I said, but this linkage of MPD and supposed sex abuse was a modern guise of that slant. "I don't believe that she is lying, and I don't believe she is insane and delusional," I testified. "I believe she has been strongly persuaded to see herself in this way by people who are promoting a particular point of view in psychiatry." I also stated that the clinicians had never tried to learn more about Donna and her family and that this failure had kept contrary evidence from their attention and led them to their erroneous judgments.

The case went to the jury, and after eight hours they returned to say they were hopelessly deadlocked: eleven members voted to acquit Mr. Smith, but one holdout, a man, later told a newspaper reporter he couldn't believe Donna could possibly "make it up." The judge dismissed the case, and the holdout juror subsequently called Donna for a date.

Although at first the prosecuting attorney planned to retry Danny Smith, the final chapter in this case came swiftly. Two weeks after the trial, the doctors at Sheppard Pratt discharged Donna to a foster home in Michigan.

Soon after she was out of the hospital and away from the continuing daily influence of the doctors and nurses on the MPD service, Donna reported that she began having doubts about her previous beliefs and especially about her claims of being abused by her father. Within a month, she called her mother and reestablished contact with the family. Her brothers had trouble forgiving her, but her parents, as could be expected, were overjoyed to be reconciled with her.

The next year the Smiths—Donna and her parents—filed suit against the Sheppard Pratt hospital and Catherine Meyers. Donna denied all her previous claims that her father had assaulted her, or that her family had taken part in any satanic rituals. She now maintained that suggestive therapy, drugs, hypnotism, and isolation led her to take on false ideas and evoked false memories, and that her doctors had encouraged her into prosecuting her father.

The hospital and doctors settled the case on the eve of the trial in 1996 for an undisclosed sum paid in damages to the Smiths. But no matter how much money they were awarded, it could not bring back the years of Donna's adolescence that were lost, nor restore completely the family's reputation to what it had been before this lengthy, painful and public ordeal.

The good thing, however, was that with this case I experienced how to work in court and what it would take to succeed. What impressed me was just how powerful a successful rebuttal in a court case could be. The Donna Smith case was eventually written up in *Esquire* magazine, was reviewed on national television, and became the first in a number of cases where the practices of the Manneristic Freudians were held up as dangerous and misguided. It was a beginning.

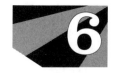

The Scope of Suspicion

O ften, when I described the recovered memory fad, I'd mention an adage of Oliver Wendell Holmes, the nineteenth-century doctor, professor of anatomy at Harvard Medical School, poet, and essayist. He wrote, "The truth is that Medicine, professedly founded on observation, is as sensitive to outside influences—political, religious, philosophical, imaginative—as is the barometer to the changes in atmospheric density."

He had in mind such eruptions as the Salem witch craze and the programs in "alternative medicine" of his own time, such as Christian Science. But the thought applies broadly. Medical practices, to this day, often rest on unstated attitudes and hidden assumptions of doctors. This is particularly true in psychiatry.

To understand the zeal and incorrigibility of the Manneristic Freudians, one needs to recognize just how fired by suspicion their imaginations were. They took their suspicious attitudes from Freud, but added their suppositions that parental betrayal of children was a common human experience and lay as a hidden generative source behind most mental disorders, such as depression and anxiety. These suspicions did not derive from empirical data but sprang from a contemporary ethos or creed.

The French philosopher Paul Ricoeur in his book *Freud and Philosophy: An Essay on Interpretation* (1970) speaks about the prestige of suspicion in modern thought. He draws attention to three key intellectual figures who, in different ways, sought to unmask and expose "realities" behind social appearances and succeeded, again in their different ways, in provoking in our culture broad-ranging suspicions about aspects of life in which trust and hope had previously and naturally resided. According to Ricoeur, "Three masters, seemingly mutually exclusive, dominate the school of suspicion: Marx, Nietzsche, and Freud."

The Mannerists followed Freud in striving to look "behind the mask of consciousness" for confirmation of their suspicions. In doing so, they brought more heavy-handed presumptions and directed all their mistrust at guardians.

During my encounters with the Manneristic Freudians, I certainly could attest to just how strong the "school of suspicion" had become in American culture. These therapists depended on it, both in winning their patients' assent when memories were "recovered" and in expecting public support when they were challenged for proof.

How widespread an attitude of suspicion had become, how fundamental it was to these practices, and how this suspicious attitude made the correction of these therapists difficult became clear to me after the Donna Smith case. That example of how unreal suspicions about parents had led to disaster had little effect, either locally in Baltimore or nationally when it was publicized. Instead of being seen as an expression of a growing professional problem in psychiatry based upon faulty assumptions, it was dismissed as a simple mistake of inexperienced practitioners. And this despite the fact that it occurred in a distinguished American psychiatric hospital and was steered throughout its course, right into the Leonardtown courtroom, by a psychiatrist identified as a national expert in multiple personality disorder.

But many similar cases were coming to courts across the country, and for those defendants the outcomes were even more disastrous. On the basis of testimony no different from what Danny Smith faced, many men (and a few women) were being found guilty of crimes they never committed and receiving punishing prison terms.

The common sense of judges, prosecuting attorneys, and juries was overwhelmed by suspicions generated in the testimony of purported victims and their psychiatric champions. The streak of paranoia represented by these suspicions even generated—as with Donna Smith—presumptions about satanic rituals and the abuse of children that were little different from the ideas in the Salem witch trials of 1692.

The pervasiveness of this climate of suspicion was also displayed in cases only slightly different from the recovered memory cases but making bigger headlines. These included the notorious McMartin preschool case in California and the Kelly Michaels case in New Jersey, in both of which young children were testifying to being abused by their teachers and caregivers in hideous ways.

The children's testimony was wilder than the adult recovered memories and included claims of deep tunneling under the earth, flying in balloons, and the most disgusting of perversions carried out by gangs of abusers. What was amazing was how these cases sprang up almost simultaneously across the country and how similar was the approach to drawing testimony from children in every one of them.

Groups of mental health workers (nurses, social workers, and psychologists) using the same obviously suggestive techniques (such as showing children "anatomically correct" dolls) and the same coercive methods of interviewing nursery school children (such as promising them candy rewards) emerged from the north and the south, the east and the west: in California with the McMartin case, in New Jersey with the Michaels case, in North Carolina with the Little Rascals case, and in Massachusetts with the Fells Acres case, to list only the ones that received the most headlines.

Draconian sentences, such as the five consecutive life terms meted out to Robert Kelly in the Little Rascals case, were imposed on those convicted. Much effort was made to gain confessions from young and innocent bystanders, like secretaries and part-time workers in the nursery school, by offering them "lighter sentences" rather than ripping them from their families and their children.

Eventually, many (but not all) of these cases were publically discredited and the mental health workers who generated them rebuked. But much damage had been done. The public can thank the 1990 article by Dorothy Rabinowitz in *Harper's* (thoroughly and brilliantly expanded upon in her *No Crueler Tyrannies: Accusation, False Witness, and Other Terrors of Our Times* [2003]) and the superb book by Stephen J. Ceci and Maggie Bruck, *Jeopardy in the Courtroom: A Scientific Analysis of Children's Testimony* (1995), for revealing the incoherence of these prosecutions, the lack of knowledge about children and suggestibility, the bandwagon effect in law enforcement and social service investigators selling each other on new notions for suggestively examining children, and the occasional bit of malice behind many of the charges.

The key to understanding these cases is, again, not that child abuse doesn't happen or that all child testimony is corrupt and untrustworthy, but that, in this period, pervasive suspicion about the good faith of people in positions of responsibility swept judgment aside. This suspicion produced what can only be considered a witch-trial atmosphere where the presumption of innocence was discarded, false testimony was credited, and standards of scientific practice (such as learning through controlled studies how young children normally approach and inspect anatomically correct dolls) were ignored.

Even as I was aware of these events and how misguided they were, it took still more experience to teach me to appreciate how suspicions built on imagination and rendered respectable by medical testimony can gain in power. I suspected something of the sort when the scandal of the Donna Smith case did nothing to alter the support for multiple personality work at Sheppard Pratt in Baltimore, but soon I met face to face with the habits of suspicion in our culture that the Mannerists count on for support.

On this occasion, I witnessed how a national newspaper dealt with a case in which I was involved. The case had seemed straightforward to most impartial observers in the courtroom, including a jury, but a bias of suspicion affected how it was ultimately reported to the public.

The accusations that generated the O'Connor case tried in Rockville, Maryland, were, I thought, a standard misuse of psychotherapy in generating false memories. David O'Connor, fifty-six, was an executive with General Electric who was accused by his daughter Kathy, age thirty-two, of abusing her multiple times.

Kathy had no memory of being a victim of sexual abuse until, when she was thirty, she began psychotherapy for depression and came to "recover" memories of being abused from infancy through adolescence by her father and some of his male friends. She was advised by lawyers to sue her father for millions of dollars.

As her case was a civil suit rather than a criminal prosecution, she, as the plaintiff, had a somewhat lessened burden of proof. She did not have to prove her accusations "beyond a reasonable doubt" but would win if a jury agreed that the "preponderance of evidence" supported her claim.

David O'Connor was tried before a jury of six, and during the several days of the trial both Kathy and her psychiatrist testified to the validity of her "recovered memories" and how the sexual abuse these "memories" brought to light explained her lifelong mental disturbances. These disturbances were far from trivial and included depressions, sexual promiscuity, drug and alcohol abuse, and aberrant personality characteristics.

I testified for the defense to the effect that many of Kathy's "memories" were just too incredible to be believed. They included multiple situations where privacy could not be guaranteed so that many witnesses should have been available, and yet she brought none to court. She was particularly insistent in "remembering" how in her infancy (twelve to eighteen months of age, before she had acquired the faculty of speech) she had been sexually assaulted and humiliated and could only scream in rage. I thought these ideas generated by psychotherapy were artifacts of the therapy itself.

I also testified that rather than due to some imagined sexual abuse from her father, Kathy's long-standing mental disorders could be more credibly attributed to the devastating effects on her psychological development of the disruption of her home life at age ten. At that most vulnerable period of childhood, her mother, now actively supporting her campaign to sue, had demanded that David leave the family home to make room for Kathy's school principal, with whom she had taken up a sexual liaison and ultimately would marry.

After only a brief deliberation, the jury found unanimously in the defendant father's favor and denied Kathy's petition for damages. This is what I had expected, given the facts in the case. But subsequent events emphasized for me how powerful suspicions can influence subsequent judgment despite those suspicions being discredited in the most public way.

On April 12, 1994, a few weeks after the O'Connor case had finished, a reporter for the *Washington Post*, Sandra Boodman, who had attended the trial, published a set of interlocking reports on the case in the *Post's* weekly health supplement. Her reports purported to be even-handed considerations of the case material but actually promoted the impression that justice had not been done to Kathy.

The articles suggested that scientific evidence existed for both the repression of memories of trauma and the accuracy of their ultimate recovery in psychotherapy. They undermined the False Memory Syndrome Foundation by identifying its members as "aggrieved" parents (using just such scare quotes to imply that their being aggrieved was unjustified) and challenged the foundation's advisory board of scientists and clinicians as lacking "much clinical experience treating trauma victims" (a strange claim to read for me, a member of that board, given that for twenty years I had been psychiatrist-in-chief at a municipal hospital in Baltimore, where violence is so frequent that two national television programs—*Homicide* and *The Wire*—sited their series in my neighborhood). Even the photographs accompanying the Boodman articles carried the implication of an injustice done by depicting a quiet Kathy O'Connor seated contemplatively at the piano as against a threatening and disreputable-appearing Peter and Pamela Freyd of the FMSF peering through wired glass like convicts.

I drew several conclusions from reading this account. If an able journalist from a nationally distinguished newspaper did not see what was wrong with recovered memory therapy despite the evidence presented in this case, and if her editors could headline her articles with the question "Are delayed memories like hers true or false?" (even though an impartial jury had rendered a clear answer to that question), then something more was at stake here than just evidence and psychiatric malpractice. We had to approach the issue in another way.

I also realized that, given the suspicions that carried prestige in the culture and found expression in Sandra Boodman's interpretations, David O'Connor had dodged a bullet. Those of us who hoped to put an end to these misdirections of clinical practice and the legal prosecutions they generated had better find a way to bring the basic claims about recovered memories to trial. We should not presume that our testimony in individual cases would be ever persuasive and eventually conclusive.

The climate of suspicion would sustain the concepts of buried sexual abuse and dominate psychiatric discourse as long as the battles were fought case by case. Regardless of the outcome of any individual case, people like Sandra Boodman—a reporter acting, I believe, in good faith—would find reasons to sustain the suspicions. Acquittals would please the defendants, convictions would please the plaintiffs, but such individual cases would not address the central issue—can we rely on uncorroborated "recovered" memories?—because that issue gets support from the "school of suspicion" and from the persistent belief that repression and recovery of traumatic memories are valid science-based psychiatric concepts to be used by victims in seeking justice.

What was needed was an "evidentiary hearing" about this issue—a hearing in which guilt and innocence of some defendant was not the main issue under debate, but rather whether a "recovered memory" can have standing as a reasonable and reliable, "stand-alone," piece of evidence to place before a jury in determining guilt and innocence.

By coincidence of timing, the question of how to adjudge scientific evidence was approached anew by the U.S. Supreme Court in an opinion rendered at the end of its 1992–93 session and thus right in the middle of our battles. The decision in *Daubert v. Merrell Dow Pharmaceuticals, Inc.*, was written by Justice Blackmun and it "assign[ed] to the trial judge the task of ensuring that an expert's testimony both rests on a reliable foundation and is relevant to the task at hand."

As the opinion further directed, an inquiry into the admissibility of any scientific concept to a trial must focus "solely" on the expert's "principles and methodology" and "not on the conclusions that they generate." To assist courts in determining the reliability of expert scientific testimony, the *Daubert* opinion offered several features to consider concerning a scientific concept. These included whether its methods had been *tested*, whether the concept had been subjected to *peer review and publication*, whether its *error rates* were known, and whether the concept itself enjoyed *widespread acceptance*.

Many in our number worried about what these so-called *Daubert* standards would mean for our efforts at challenging recovered memories, since they replaced the old test—the so-called *Frye* test—that had stood since 1923 and where scientific evidence was admissible in court only if it had gained "general acceptance." But I and several others thought that the greater specificity of the *Daubert* approach would help us in an evidentiary hearing, given that the issue would turn on whether recovered memories in and of themselves are accurate testimonies. We had already demonstrated errors based on them and presumed that the error rate would climb with more study.

We repeatedly said that we were not claiming that it was impossible to forget a trauma. Likewise, we were not claiming that a course of long-term psychotherapy would never uncover new facts that had not been appreciated for their implications by a patient at the start.

We knew full well that things can be forgotten and later remembered and that cases to that effect could be adduced. But we also knew that the forgetting in those cases usually had simple explanations. These included most of the ordinary reasons people forget things: the simple fading of memories with time, the misunderstanding of an event when it happened and especially if it occurred so early in life it fell into the period of infantile amnesia, an accompanying head injury that thwarted perception and consolidation of memories, or the common response of suppressing conscious dwelling on an event and then misconstruing that lack of attention as an actual loss of the memory of that event. These explanations would not demand the invoking of mental mechanisms so esoteric, cryptic, or mysterious as repression or dissociation.

The normal ways of forgetting and remembering not only would explain cases better than repression, but the very fact that these ways of forgetting and remembering occur would require psychiatrists to use a standard and coherent method of assessing a patient claiming a new memory, a method that I'll describe later in this book. It was this method of assessment that the Manneristic Freudians, when promoting their beliefs in sexual abuse, put aside and that many reporters of "forgetting and recovery" cases failed to demand.

To put the issue in the simplest and clearest terms, I hoped that through a *Daubert* hearing we would demonstrate that the sentence we had met at every turn—"The ordinary response to atrocities is to banish them from consciousness"—was false. (That brook-no-contradiction line opened Judith Herman's book *Trauma and Recovery* [1992] and was scripture to our opponents.)

We hold to the contrary (and with psychological and social scientific support) that the "ordinary" response to atrocity is remembering it. An absence of memory "ordinarily" will mean the absence of trauma and should not encourage the use of suggestive techniques to overcome some supposed resistance to remembering. Those techniques, we were claiming, were not new and better ways of assessing the mentally ill, but were products of a school of suspicion misdirecting psychiatric practice and poisoning the culture.

To gain judicial support for our point of view would suffice to render the presentation of a "recovered memory" in court—or anywhere else, for that matter, such as the newspapers and television—untenable unless other, independent validating observations accompanied it. Most "recovered memories" would be seen for what they are: beliefs rather than memories. They should be studied so as to learn how they came to pass, by considering the circumstances around their appearance and what significance they might have in a patient's life history, experiences, and assumptions.

For me, that would be wonderful. It would teach in a public arena just how psychotherapists must approach the beliefs and other attitudes and assumptions of patients. Better care and service from psychiatry to patients, families, and the public would certainly ensue.

We were put to the *Daubert* test in the spring of 1995, when the superior court in New Hampshire called for an evidentiary hearing combining two cases of importance to us: *The State of New Hampshire v. Joel Hungerford* and *The State of New Hampshire v. John Morahan.* Judge William J. Groff would adjudicate.

Mr. Hungerford had been charged with the repeated rape of his now twenty-seven-year-old daughter during her childhood. Mr. Morahan, a junior high school teacher, had been charged with raping one of his students, now in her late twenties, when she was thirteen. Both women had had no recollection of the abuse prior to entering psychotherapy and had "recovered" memories of these purported crimes over the course of that therapy.

These two cases were seen as similar by the New Hampshire Superior Court and prompted a similar demand. Before the cases could be sent to trial, the court ruled that the state must prove the evidentiary worth of "repressed memories" according to the *Daubert* standards.

The state prosecutors would have to show, for example, that psychological experts generally accept the process by which "memories" are summoned into consciousness and that the errors of fact in memories so summoned were so few that the memories would be sufficient in themselves rather than need confirmatory evidential support. Such questions would need to be addressed before the women could testify to their "recollections" in trial.

This hearing produced a historic confrontation between those who believed in the validity of recovered memories and the soundness of processes used to evoke them and those, like me, who saw the recovered memory therapies as deeply flawed and ultimately dangerous to all concerned—patients and families. I flew to Manchester, New Hampshire, to testify, as did my comrades-in-arms Elizabeth Loftus and psychiatrist James Hudson of the McLean Hospital in Boston.

I was on the witness stand for most of a day under direct and cross-examination. I talked mostly about how the issue of recovering traumatic memories, far from being generally accepted, had divided psychiatrists into wrangling camps.

I emphasized how socially dangerous the concept of repression was in that no one could be safe from prosecution if it was employed without confirming evidence. I based that conclusion on the following logic: First, it had proven impossible to demonstrate repression under controlled conditions; second, an accusation based on an indemonstrable mechanism (rather than on tangible evidence) would be irrefutable; hence, if no one can defend against an indemonstrable, irrefutable charge, no one was safe from prosecution should these ideas about memory and trauma be accepted.

To demonstrate just how far this concept of memory repression had progressed, I reviewed the reception of popular books that had become best sellers. These included not only *Sybil*, where "forgotten" sexual abuse was first linked to multiple personality disorder, but also *Michelle Remembers* (1980), which proposed the existence of satanic cults abusing children throughout our nation, and *Communion: A True Story* (1987), which describes sexual abuse supposedly committed by aliens from space.

I tried to connect all of these ideas and expressions to the school of suspicion that I saw as one of the legacies of Sigmund Freud. I pointed out how Freud's suspicions of human motivations began with efforts to persuade his neurotic patients that they had been abused but how he ultimately abandoned that tack—mostly because even he could not believe the amount of child abuse his theory implied, as even members of his own family would be implicated—and he searched for and came up with his idea of infantile sexuality to sustain his suspicions that human nature and society are fundamentally at odds.

If I went too far along these lines, Judge Groff would draw me back. Occasionally he had to remind me that in court, unlike in the clinic, there is little time for or interest in academic speculating—the judicial process is serious, focused, and laden with consequence.

The hearing also permitted strong advocates of the recovered memory movement to be heard. They included Bessel van der Kolk, then on the faculty at Harvard Medical School; Jon Conte, a professor of social work from the University of Washington; and Daniel Brown, a psychologist from the Massachusetts Mental Health Center.

They claimed that good evidence supported the concept of memory retrieval, even with hypnotic induction, and they attested to the validity of memories of abuse generated through such means. But when they were cross-examined, they admitted that some of the claims of abuse made by at least one of the women involved in the New Hampshire cases were "unlikely."

The hearing was long, but the wait for judgment was longer. Its duration rested on the thoroughness with which Judge Groff approached his task. Not only did his final judgment go to the heart of our contention about the recovery of memory, but it enunciated in clear terms the problem of error in this matter.

He explained that any claim of memory loss after trauma is first a scientific claim (i.e., this is how the human mind functions) before it is a clinical claim (i.e., this patient can be understood as one who repressed the memory of her sexual abuse by the accused). The law must strive to ensure that scientific ideas still under debate are not presented to lay juries as if they were settled matters of fact—even if and when some clinicians do use the idea in practice. He also noted that scientific and clinical debate over these issues obviously existed, given the strong testimony from well-qualified people presented at the hearing itself.

Judge Groff not only ordered that evidentiary standards be satisfied, but he also added several other criteria to be considered before recovered memories were presented in the courtroom because, he wrote, of the "great possibility of suggestiveness in therapy."

In particular, he held that courts considering these matters of belief over abuse look to (1) the age of the witness at the time of the alleged abuse, (2) the length of time between the alleged event and the recovery of the memory, (3) the presence or absence of objective, verifiable corroborative evidence of the remembered abusive event, and (4) the circumstances attendant to the recovery of the memory.

Judge Groff concluded that in the Hungerford and Morahan cases, the testimony of the accusing women could not be admitted because the foundations of their testimony—based as it was on "recovered memories," on the assumption that trauma produces repression of memory, and on the means used by therapists in these cases to "recover" the memories—were flawed in themselves and had not gained general acceptance in the psychological and psychiatric fields.

He also explained how he saw this kind of testimony—when not confirmed—to be dangerous to society and to the judicial process:

> Being labeled a child abuser [is] one of the most loathsome labels in society ... with grave physical, emotional, professional, and personal ramifications. Harm caused by misdiagnosis extends beyond the accused parent [to] devastate the whole family. Society also suffers because false accusations cast doubt on true claims of abuse and undermine efforts to identify and eradicate sexual abuse.

He explicitly noted:

> A therapist owes an accused parent a duty of care in the treatment of an adult patient for sexual abuse where the therapist (or the patient acting on the encouragement, recommendation, or instruction of the therapist) takes public action concerning the accusation. In such instances the social utility of detecting and punishing sexual abusers and maintaining the breadth of treatment choices for patients is outweighed by the substantial risk of severe harm to falsely accused parents, the family unit, and society.

How I cheered his opinion. "A Daniel come to judgment!" I could shout. This judicial decision not only supported my definitions of coherent psychiatric practices to the full, but it also spoke to the problems that the overly suspicious could generate in our culture.

Yet this decision was much more than just a vindication of my teaching. It particularly vindicated the FMSF. Things might have worked out in the long run as they did anyway, but "the long run" would have been grim. The FMSF garnered attention about how people were being mistreated and encouraged scientific challenges to the concept of repression. These efforts speeded the process of refutation, spared many potential victims, and exemplified how a school of suspicion can be thwarted.

I thought about the old witch trials that had occurred only about sixty miles away from the Manchester courtroom. Those poor folks never had, and certainly could have used, such an FMSF-like advocacy group to attack the attitudes of suspicion and credulity that characterized that culture.

After *Hungerford* and *Morahan*, accused abusers in recovered memory cases could ask for—and have a reasonable expectation of receiving—an evidentiary hearing challenging the validity of recovered memories like the ones in these cases. And it was not long coming, for I was drawn into another *Daubert* hearing in which, if it were possible, even more was at stake for a defendant.

This adventure began with a letter I received from a Jack Quattrocchi, who had been convicted and had already served twenty-five months of a sixty-year sentence for, so it was claimed, repeatedly abusing the daughter of his onetime girlfriend. Quattrocchi, a fifty-four-year-old Vietnam veteran, was obviously a brave man: he had refused to admit to crimes he didn't commit, even though the judge had told him that such an admission would reduce his sentence to a "more manageable" eight years.

Only now the Rhode Island Supreme Court ordered him retried, citing the *Hungerford/Morahan* decision in New Hampshire. Quattrocchi, the court said, was entitled to an evidentiary hearing to determine whether the accuser's claims of remembering her abuse were based on scientifically trustworthy practices and thus properly admitted to trial as evidence against him.

The hearing eventually was launched in March 1998 before Judge Edward C. Clifton of the Rhode Island Superior Court, and I appeared in Quattrocchi's defense at the request of his attorney, Chris Barden, who would prove to be an intrepid fighter against recovered memory claims. The hearing would determine whether the prosecutors who had previously convicted Quattrocchi would drop the case and allow him to walk free. If they were permitted again to bring before an impressionable jury a tearful young woman who had undergone years of emotionally evocative, memory-"enhancing" psychotherapy, that jury would likely return him to what essentially amounted to a life sentence in a Rhode Island prison.

These considerations greatly troubled me. My previous experience (I had now appeared in several other cases), far from making me confident as a witness, had taught me how luck can influence the outcome in court. I'd learned that it helps to have the truth on your side when facing a judge and jury, but that truth does not always win the day.

I was shaken by the responsibilities I would be asked to carry here. If my testimony was clumsy or I failed to stand up against prosecutorial cross-examination, this man might spend the rest of his days in a jail cell and I'd be haunted by the vision.

As I flew up to Providence, I thought, "This is a young man's game." With stakes so high, old guys like me (I was nearing sixty-seven) might not be able to sustain the energy or fortitude needed to beat back a dedicated, aggressive opponent. I was braced by the example of Quattrocchi's own bravery in refusing to accept a plea bargain, but I knew I must muster every resource of skill and energy I had to prevail.

The other side was impressive. Although a number of the usual experts for recovered memory, such as Daniel Brown, whom I had met at the *Hungerford/Morahan* hearing, were due to appear, also on the list was the thoughtful Paul Applebaum, then chairman of the Department of Psychiatry at the University of Massachusetts Medical School, a devout Orthodox Jew, and soon to be president of the American Psychiatric Association.

Given the seriousness with which Dr. Applebaum customarily approached all his responsibilities and his undoubted study of the evidence in light of the *Hungerford/Morahan* decision, I wondered and worried as to whether I could rebut what he would say. It had to count heavily in the eyes of a judge that such a sincere and distinguished man was prepared to help rob Quattrocchi of life by entombing him in a Rhode Island prison.

I did, however, have some definite advantages. The evidence, at least as I saw it, was remarkably clear. Written records demonstrated that the young woman accusing Quattrocchi had been slow to agree that he had abused her and for months had resisted powerful psychological and family pressure to produce "memories."

On anything like a reasonable reading of this evidence, I found it hard to fathom how anyone would believe that this young woman was now to be believed. And yet the prosecuting attorneys were convinced that Quattrocchi was a guilty man who deserved to be punished—and punished severely.

Their stance surprised me as much as other aspects of this case because I felt a kinship with these guys. Providence has, like my hometown of Lawrence, Massachusetts, many Irish-American prosecutors—people I've known since childhood as both tough-minded about life and fair about justice. Bright, articulate, skeptical almost to the point of cynicism, they would usually identify as smoke and mirrors much of what passes as reason in psychiatric practice.

That the chief prosecutor in this case—with his New England accent, Irish visage, and general air of no-nonsense—would believe the evidence I'd seen and be ready to nail Quattrocchi with it showed me that the tsunami of suspicion in our culture could sweep away even the sturdiest breed. It could persuade this man to bank on practices that were coercive on their face because they supported belief in hidden trauma.

The psychiatric facts were straightforward and really not in dispute. The accuser was an unstable teenager who had been in treatment for years combating brittle emotions, explosive rages, and depression. She lived with her mother, who had for several years cohabited with Jack Quattrocchi. The mother herself suffered from depression and alcohol problems and, embittered by her breakup with Quattrocchi, had been the first to suggest to her daughter that perhaps Quattrocchi had sexually abused her.

One of the reasons she adduced was that Jack had maintained a friendship with the daughter even to the point of helping pay for her schooling. Quattrocchi, in reply, claimed that he had come to love the girl like a child of his own when he lived with the mother. This continuing but paternal affection prompted him to offer financial help for her education.

The mother reported her beliefs to the accuser's therapist, a nurse practicing psychotherapy, and as the notes reveal, without a moment's reflection on the possible bias of the source, the therapist adopted them, writing, "I am assuming, as is her mother, that he [Quattrocchi] sexually abused her." Subsequent notes, however, also demonstrate that the young patient specifically and repeatedly said, "Nothing ever happened. He was like my father."

Nonetheless, the therapist wrote in the case notes available for all to read that the specific goal of her treatment of this young woman "has been to help her try to re-create those memories." Again, though (and nine months into this process), the therapist's records describe how the patient "repeatedly states 'I really don't remember' but I [the therapist] do not believe this to be so. States 'he is like my Dad, he couldn't have done anything bad to me.' Plan to continue working towards dealing with abuse issue."

With the therapist continuing this "plan," the patient eventually began to have "memories." As soon as she said anything about "remembering abuse," the therapist reported Quattrocchi to the Department of Child Services and the prosecution began.

The therapist continued to dig by encouraging the patient to "try to remember" even more. The patient's accusations began to expand. Ultimately they would encompass rape, threats of violence, and the like—none of which was "remembered" until long into therapy.

In the process of "remembering" and "describing" these incidents, the patient collapsed emotionally and her capacities to continue in school or work were lost. She required several hospitalizations for severe depression and suicidal thoughts. The therapist interpreted these worsening symptoms as "only natural," given what the patient had come to "realize." This problematic, artful psychological interpretation would support the prosecutor's view of her as a suffering victim.

Despite all that was at stake—the life of a member of the community previously considered worthy—neither the therapist nor the police made any attempt to confirm or refute the "memories." They did not bring in another psychiatrist to look at the evidence and treatment plan, as standards of care would call for when the patient is getting worse despite months of "therapy." A second opinion might have cleared away the blinding emotional baggage that this case was accumulating with everyone.

Everyone in law enforcement in Providence seemed to agree that if a mentally disturbed teenager changed her long-repeated claims from "nothing ever happened" to "he raped me," the last claim should be prosecuted without question.

I recognized a paradoxical response of therapists working to recover "memories." The long period of patient resistance to the idea of sex abuse does not lead them to doubt their suspicions any more than the surrender of patients to persistent questioning leads them to wonder about suggestion. Rather, the repeated experience of this sequence of events—long resistance, ultimate concurrence—made therapists progressively more certain of both their skill at identifying abuse victims and the power of repression to hold recollections of abuse at bay.

In the beginning, they see the patients as "in denial" and later as "open" to reality. Such is the therapists' world, where words and concepts justify their sequence of judgments.

At the hearing, I testified that the therapy notes revealed many instances of leading and suggestive questions. They also revealed bias on the part of the mother and therapist—a bias that created the suspicion about sexual abuse and about Quattrocchi specifically. I identified the treatment, which had led to Quattrocchi's indictment, as far from standard—indeed, I considered the approaches used with this patient to be travesties of psychotherapy. "Believe the victim" and "Believe the therapists" tended to be slogans that were running hand in hand and unchallenged because they matched what people suspected. No one was looking dispassionately at the facts or the treatment methods.

I said that when psychotherapy brings to public attention matters such as sexual abuse, then the suggestive nature and limits to confidence tied to such treatment need to be appreciated. That would dispel any mystery and direct the next steps in assessment. These considerations were overlooked and neglected in this case.

When pressed by the prosecutors in cross-examination on this point, I closed my testimony by reviewing a highly regarded, recently published article on the remembering of sexual abuse by subjects who were on record in emergency rooms as having been sexually abused in years past.[1] This article by Linda Meyer Williams was being put forward as proof that people "repress" their experience of sexual abuse. She showed that some 38 percent of the subjects failed to report an abuse that the investigators knew had occurred, and 12 percent any abuse at all.

I identified my reasons for challenging an implicit interpretation that these results reveal the "repression" of sex abuse memories. First, there were no "controls" (no effort to discern whether the failures to report would have been similar if the subjects had had some accident, rather than been sexually abused). Second, many of the subjects reported multiple occasions of abuse but not the particular occasion at issue (and thus they may have forgotten the specific occasion amid a mass of dreadful experiences). Third, many of the subjects were under the age of five at the time of the abuse (thus subject to infantile amnesia). Fourth, and most telling, the investigator did not probe the subjects for their recollection, and thus she could not say whether some of those failing to report were simply unwilling to talk about what they had found embarrassing.

For all that a clinician could agree that this method would identify some forgetfulness, it could not support the concept that repression comes commonly with sex abuse.

In the end, I came to see that my testimony—to the effect that the treatment this young woman received and from which her accusations emerged did not meet standards of care and was not at all what psychotherapy should be—was not decisive in this hearing. Nor did Dr. Applebaum's defense of the concept of repression, and the therapies used to recover "memories" of trauma, carry the day.

What ultimately led Judge Clifton to throw out the accusations against Quattrocchi was the testimony of the scientists: Elizabeth Loftus and Richard Ofshe.

The prosecutors had argued that the *Daubert* criteria should be "relaxed" in this and other abuse cases because of the subjective character of data in psychiatry and psychology that made many theories hard to "verify scientifically." But the judge listened closely to Loftus and Ofshe as they described detailed experiments they had conducted on how memory works and can be distorted. This convinced him that scientific knowledge challenged the memories that the prosecution rested upon.

He heard Richard Ofshe discuss his ideas that the claims for repression offered in this case were actually for a kind of "robust" repression that goes far beyond what even the Freudian psychoanalysts claimed about repression. Ofshe pointed out how a claim that all knowledge of an event could be driven from awareness within minutes of its happening had no previous foundation in psychological science and was not supported by either current psychological studies or the neuroscience of memory. People may not remember all the particular details of a traumatic and frightening experience, but they certainly remember the gist of the event unless something like a head injury renders them unconscious.

Elizabeth Loftus drew out her studies on how memories are highly "constructive" mental features that rest on three interrelated functions or faculties—an encoding, storing, and retrieval function. The encoding faculty permits humans to enter as memories those events that seem salient when they happen. These encoded memories then pass through the short-term storing faculty (where they may die away unless they have more than immediate salience) to reach long-term storage. There they can be distorted and changed by new memories but will gradually fade if not recalled. The retrieval faculty recovers a memory of past events for consciousness, but not as a perfect replication of the original events: it will often modify what is remembered so that it fits expectations and other confounding factors at the time of retrieval.

Memories are thus, Loftus explained, open to many transformations at several levels—encoding, storage, and retrieval—so that not only are most memories not a direct match of the original events, but many things can be "recovered" that never happened.

She provided a number of examples from her own research where she had suggested to perfectly normal subjects—subtly and with supportive collaborators—that in their past they had experienced some distressful event, such as being lost or having had some minor injury. Although all of them said at the initiation that they had no memory of such an event, many during an interview weeks later not only "recovered the memory" in a form similar to what Loftus had "implanted" but were so convinced such an event had happened they added details to the story.

Drawing on this laboratory experience, Loftus noted how the approach of the therapist in the Quattrocchi case—where repeated questions carrying the suspicions of abuse bombarded the patient so as to help her "remember"—was similar to the approach she had used to instill false memories in her subjects. That eventually the patient agreed and even elaborated on the suggestions was very typical, Loftus said.

Because this was an evidentiary *Daubert* hearing, Judge Clifton didn't have to choose a side in the ongoing debate between scientists, clinicians, and lawyers. He had only to establish that a valid debate among informed experts existed. And that's what he did, eventually writing a clear opinion where he stated, "The areas of consensus regarding repressed recollection remain greatly clouded by continuing and overriding division and discrepancy within the applicable fields."

With this decision, the prosecution collapsed. Quattrocchi was free, I could breathe, and we all had splendid scientific associates to thank.

My colleagues and I had won again. We had together confronted what had been a travesty of justice and had overcome it. But I remained shaken by this nearest miss with disaster and with how suspicions of Quattrocchi's motivations, tainted by malice, had been able to run riot when given the trappings of "therapy."

There was more here than just a foolish therapist to explain. Something in the culture itself—some devotion to suspicion—had led ordinarily careful people to abandon judgment and join in what amounted to a persecution of Quattrocchi.

Reminded again of what Oliver Wendell Holmes had said about how imaginative influences can affect medicine, I began to attend to this remarkable social phenomenon—a commitment to suspicion over trust, with psychotherapy as its instrument—even as the legal battles moved to the next stage. I could see that with the *Hungerford/Morahan* and *Quattrocchi* decisions, I and my colleagues had gained some vindication for coherent psychiatry and psychotherapy, especially in arenas as fraught with confusion as memory and child abuse.

We had defended several people and rescued them from persecution. But to stop the persecution elsewhere, what we had done for defendants would have to be done for plaintiffs, as "payback time" in court had arrived for the Manneristic Freudians.

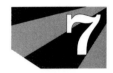

Moving from
Defense to Offense

An adversarial courtroom often must accomplish for psychotherapists what an autopsy room does for physicians and surgeons: display to them in the most forceful fashion just how they went wrong—hence, my interest in the cases that followed the *Daubert* hearings. They were brought by patients and families claiming that recovered memory therapists had misled and injured them.

The allegations revealed an important and interesting fact about these cases. Two distinctive groups of practitioners propelled them.

One group was large and made up of relatively incompetent therapists from a mixed bag of clinical disciplines. The other was small and consisted of a tightly knit faction of psychiatrists, the Manneristic Freudians: arguably competent but fixed on their claims and theories and closed to criticism.

The lack of skill or serious professionalism in the first group should not blind anyone to the essential responsibility of the second group for the catastrophes that ensued. As I will attempt to explain in this chapter, the far-reaching influence of the second group in psychiatry sustains the practices of the first and hinders efforts to stop them.

The incompetent were drawn mostly from the ranks of nurses, social workers, and counselors (although some psychiatrists were found among them). They usually acted in solo practice and were eager to treat patients in ways they saw as "up to date." They certainly learned from the Mannerists by attending the "continuing education programs" the latter ran and occasionally consulted with them over cases or made referrals to them. They relied, however, on the authority of the Mannerists for their support.

In their treatments, they would regularly push books such as *The Courage to Heal* (1988) on their patients to advance their treatment plans. They enthusiastically proclaimed the slogans they found in those books, slogans like "If you think you were abused and your life shows the symptoms, then you were." They frequently blundered into trouble and lost control of their cases.

The leading Manneristic Freudians are psychiatrists. They hold satisfactory educational credentials. They work in major centers, where they exert considerable influence and direct programs on "Trauma," "MPD," and "Memory" that draw attention and support. They often have strong personalities, firm commitments, and energy, along with organizational skills. They bring to their institutions certain benefits, such as a profitable flow of patients referred from a wide area. These characteristics and feats help them advance to positions in their institutions where they face little challenge and less scrutiny until things go radically awry, as they occasionally do.

I learned much about the two kinds of practitioners through functioning as an expert witness in two remarkable malpractice cases. These revealed distinctions that helped me understand just why the problem of malpractice among recovered memory therapists was so widespread and why it would be difficult to confront.

A good example of the incompetent practitioner was the psychiatrist Dr. Kenneth Olson, who treated Nadean Cool in Appleton, Wisconsin. This case came to trial and I testified in it in early 1997. Nadean Cool sued Olson for the negligent use of hypnosis, implanting false memories of traumatic abuse, and mischaracterizing her as someone with multiple personality disorder.

The case can be traced back to July 1986, when Dr. Olson, a newly minted psychiatrist, moved to Appleton and brought to town his fascination with multiple personality disorder, along with his enthusiasm for hypnosis. Prior to his arrival, there were no MPD patients in Appleton, but soon he was discovering them. Nadean Cool was one of many others—several of whom would eventually sue him for similar malpractice.

Ms. Cool was a nursing assistant on the psychiatric services of St. Elizabeth's Hospital when Dr. Olson first arrived. She had in the past suffered from bulimia and alcohol abuse but was now distressed by domestic troubles with her fourteen-year-old daughter. She referred herself to this new doctor in town, Dr. Olson, in November 1986. His evaluation turned immediately away from her contemporary complaints to attend to what might lie hidden in the patient's early life.

The doctor failed to consider other aspects of her history, such as her career and family life. He made no attempt to gather a sense of her personality or current situation through a meeting with her husband, and he never contacted her former psychiatrist to learn what had helped her previously. Rather, on their first meeting, Dr. Olson told her that she was suffering from post-traumatic stress disorder (PTSD) of long standing and proposed that she begin what is best described as a "cathartic" therapy.

This therapy would turn on encouraging her to remember mistreatments from her parents and siblings during her childhood and adolescence and to express as vigorously as possible the feelings of anger and distress that she had and "still must have" about the past. She was to "try to remember" as much as she could and then vent the feelings that the recall produced—all to relieve her PTSD.

Within a month, Olson began using hypnosis to bring forth more memories and introduced the idea that she was suffering from MPD. With this treatment, though, the patient's symptoms of depression and discouragement worsened rather than improved, and the first of what would be multiple hospitalizations began. Eventually, using almost daily hypnotic sessions, Olson came to explain to Cool that she had 120 separate and distinct personalities—including those of children, adults, angels, even a duck—as a reaction to severe childhood abuse that she had "repressed."

He eventually had her believing that she had been sexually abused by her father and brother, had been forced into an abortion, and had witnessed the murder of an eight-year-old childhood friend within a satanic cult and been repeatedly raped at cult gatherings. The therapy sessions increased in frequency to daily visits and occasional marathon sessions of ten to fifteen hours, during which emotional outbursts were encouraged. These sessions were long because they consisted of calling up every "personality"—each of which had to speak of the horrors suffered that this and only this "alter" could remember.

Ultimately, as symptoms burgeoned and the patient sank into a state of suicidal depression, Dr. Olson came to think that something super-natural must explain her condition. He wondered whether the patient was "possessed" by evil spirits from the satanic cult. If so, these "spirits" were "fighting the therapy" and needed to be exorcised according to the rite of exorcism of the Roman Catholic Church.

When he could not get the local priest or bishop to agree with his proposal, he began exorcisms on his own in one of the hospital's operating rooms. Adding to the chaos, Dr. Olson brought a fire extinguisher with him during these exorcisms because he thought that with the expulsion of the demons the patient might burst into flames.

Ultimately, after five years of treatment during which she steadily wors-ened into a condition of chronic suicidal depression, Nadean Cool was transferred to another psychiatrist because Dr. Olson was moving from Wisconsin. Her new psychiatrist followed the motto of all competent physi-cians when facing a confusing clinical problem: "Keep it simple, stupid," which translates into "simplicity above all."

He didn't challenge the previous treatments, but stopped all hypnotic activities, gradually cut back and eliminated the sedatives, and encour-aged Cool to think about her present situation and how she could recover her previous interests in home life and work, rather than concentrate on her past. Her moods promptly improved, her preoccupations fell away, and her "alters" disappeared. Within a few months the only problem that remained was her profound dismay over the long periods of sickness and disability she suffered and the burdens that she had imposed on her family.

When the case eventually came to court, I testified to the many interactive errors of omission and commission evident from the case records—errors that revealed a fundamental incompetence on the part of Dr. Olson. He had omitted any effort to understand the patient's current social and psychological difficulties, but right from the start had encouraged her to search her past for the sources of her present troubles. He made no effort to consider alternatives, but believed that hidden past traumas were the sole possible explanations of her distress.

He put great emphasis on hypnosis in his treatment and emphasized to the patient that she would find in hypnotic trances the ability to "call up" memories he "knew" were there. Over time her recollections were shaped by what he encouraged, and she followed his lead in seeking satanic cult memories. All efforts of the patient to withdraw from these ideas he described as aspects of "denial."

When she worsened relentlessly, the doctor lost all judgment and turned to religious rather than natural explanations of this case. He failed to rethink his diagnosis and his treatments as the patient's condition spun out of control. Her prompt recovery when a new psychiatrist took up a coherent approach confirmed these views of the case and its mismanagement.

Not surprisingly, given the absence of any evidence that Nadean Cool had been abused and the recorded evidence of Dr. Olson's extreme, bizarre, and unprofessional methods, his insurance company agreed to settle out of court before the trial was complete. The Cools received $2.4 million from the company and the State of Wisconsin, which supports the malpractice insurance for physicians.

This example of the ideas and actions of the incompetent therapist could be replicated in many other cases. The nurse-practitioner in the Quattrocchi case provided another typical example.

But if the problem with MPD and recovered memories was simply incompetence, it would not have been so widespread and difficult to remedy. For the problem to persist so broadly, it needed well-tended conceptual roots. These came to light in the case of Patty Burgus, where an established MPD expert working within a major academic medical center also faced a legal challenge to his methods of thought and practice.

In 1997, Patty Burgus sued Dr. Bennett G. Braun and the Rush–Presbyterian–St. Luke's Medical Center in Chicago—a hospital center affiliated with the Rush University Medical Center, where Braun—a psychiatrist of some distinction in his mid-fifties—was a faculty member in the Department of Psychiatry.

Braun had Freudian training but, impressed by the ideas about MPD promoted by Cornelia Wilbur, he joined other enthusiasts in reawakening interest in MPD in the late 1970s. He was a founder of the International Society for the Study of Multiple Personality and Dissociation that emerged from this group and that, with its journal *Dissociation*, permitted its members to confer with one another and then claim their ideas had received "peer review."[1]

In 1987, Braun opened the first in-patient hospital service at the Rush–Presbyterian–St. Luke's Medical Center dedicated to the treatment of patients with multiple personality disorder and named it the Dissociative Disorders Unit. There, with a staff of nurses and social workers and resident psychiatrists, he treated many patients for MPD and repressed memories. He used this center to teach others, and his influence spread beyond the medical college. His center became a referral center in the Midwest.

His authority at Rush University Medical Center grew. He was given teaching time with medical students during their psychiatric rotations so as to inform them of the nature of his work and how they needed to know about the existence of satanic worship and ritual abuse in America today. The other members of the Department of Psychiatry apparently agreed with him and were convinced that his program was fundamentally an advance over the classical Freudian approach. But the history of the Burgus case reveals just what was happening on his unit.

Patty Burgus came from Iowa where she developed a severe depressive disorder after the birth of her second child. This depression proved resistant to treatment, and her therapist in Des Moines came to believe—in part through the teachings of Braun—that she suffered from MPD. This diagnostic decision launched a program of treatment that would last for six years—from 1986 to 1992. After some months, she was referred to the Braun group in Chicago, where most of her treatment then proceeded, she being one of the first patients to populate the new Dissociative Disorders Unit.

Braun and his staff concurred with the Iowa diagnosis of MPD. But Braun decided as well that, given the severity of her depression, Burgus was likely a victim of the most severe kind of sexual and physical abuse of the sort produced by a satanic cult. Indeed he thought she was probably still under the control of Satanists in Iowa.

He told her of his opinions and how the mind works to repress the memory of severe trauma. He indicated that the only way she could recover would be by submitting to the services of his unit, where with hypnosis and group therapies more of the details of the abuse and its contemporary significance would come to light. No alternative diagnostic possibilities were discussed with her or her husband, no different treatment programs were laid out, and no warning of complications of the treatment were given to her.

She was kept under continuous treatment by the Dissociative Disorders Unit for two years. She was frequently hypnotized to help her remember and then given sedation with benzodiazepine sedatives, such as Xanax, for her emotional reactions as "memories" emerged. She was encouraged to draw up more memories by interacting in the daily group therapy with other patients who also believed they had MPD and were victims of abuse, including satanic ritual abuse.

As the treatment proceeded, Burgus and the staff came to believe she had more than three hundred personalities, all actively affecting her thoughts, moods, and behaviors—and all tied in some way to the ritual abuse she allegedly had suffered and banished from consciousness with repression, dissociation, and multiple personality formation.

Braun's staff developed more and more wild ideas about the patient's background and the nature of her abuse. The hospital records are remarkably frank about these matters and bring home the lack of judgment and self-criticism rampant on the unit. Here is a verbatim segment of the family history section of the Burgus clinical notes in the Rush medical records: "On both sides of her family there is a long history, dating back to the 15th C. in Croatia, of Satanic Cult involvement at the highest level (Royal Blood Line)."

Consider for a moment the implications of this recorded contention about Burgus's family history. First, it presumes the truth of what is now recognized as one of the two great myths that sprang from the Middle Ages—belief in satanic worship (the other is the "blood libel" against the Jews). Second, it presumes that this woman from Des Moines could link herself to a backwater region of Europe at a time predating the voyages of Christopher Columbus. Finally, it presumes that one can trace a genealogical line and specify the identity of individuals within an ancestral pool some twenty generations in the past.

Medical science? Nonsense. We all know that any person's ancestral pool twenty generations back is huge. It amounts to 2 to the 20th power, or 1,048,576 people. Members of the psychiatric staff at Rush—a university center presumably alive to the world of fact—believed they could identify from amid that throng of ancestors a particular group of Satanists, and they encouraged Patty Burgus to believe that she was still a part of this group's successful effort to carry a "transgenerational" satanic cult into present day Iowa.

As Braun and the staff at Rush incorporated these suggestions into their treatment of her, Burgus eventually produced "memories" of the activities of the satanic cult right there in Des Moines during her childhood. She claimed to have watched the traditional rituals of the cult—black masses and other ceremonies during which babies were slaughtered and their flesh eaten while older children, including Burgus, were sexually molested.

Braun and his staff believed that the cult had powers over Burgus. They told her it could turn her into a "killing machine" responsive to coded messages, such as depicted in Richard Condon's *The Manchurian Candidate*. All communications with her family in Iowa were stopped when she received a Valentine card from one of them. The staff told Burgus that the color red in the card (rather common in Valentines) might well be a way that the cult leaders in Iowa were striving to "trigger" her "pre-programmed" murderous impulses.

The belief that the cult might generate various forms of mischief led the doctors to admit Burgus's two sons—ages four and five—to the children's unit, where they were kept in treatment and subjected to their own disturbing therapy sessions. They were shown and taught how handcuffs, knives, and revolvers might be employed to hurt children. They, like their mother, were kept in the hospital for several years so as to protect them and keep them from becoming "recruits" in the cult.

Dr. Braun's prescriptions and practices with Burgus required and received the collaborative support of many of his colleagues and staff at Rush. They helped hypnotize her and taught her about satanic cults by showing her versions of the "witch calendar" so as to explain why special protections were provided at Halloween and the various solstices and equinoxes, when "Satan's helpers" exert more of their diabolic energies.

All of this, along with the continuing use of sedation, kept Burgus in a state of terror. She was told that there would be more to discover if she "tried still harder to remember" her past. As particular fears of her own began to emerge, they encouraged her to look into them with all seriousness.

For example, she had her husband bring hamburger meat to the hospital from Des Moines so that the laboratory could search it for human tissue as evidence of the cannibalism that might be active at home. As far as the records show, this strange episode was the only effort made by the staff at Rush to check the likelihood of an ongoing criminal cult in Iowa. No one thought it worthwhile to call the Des Moines police because many in the staff believed that "the Satanists would surely have infiltrated the police."

The health insurance companies continued to pay for these prolonged hospitalizations of Burgus and her children. Their psychiatric advisors had no way of challenging her treatment, given that the diagnosis of MPD was legitimized by *DSM-III*, and in the Chicago community Dr. Braun was credited as *the* expert in its identification and management.

Eventually, after years in this program and the severe mental distress it evoked in her, Burgus and her husband began to wonder about her treatment. They went back to Des Moines and visited all the places where the cult abuse, the child murders, the witches' Sabbaths, and the like were to have taken place. Not surprisingly, they found no tangible evidence for such activities; no bones, no altars, no graves, no remnants of anything untoward was to be found.

Burgus then stayed in Des Moines, and without the continuing hypnotic treatments and the sedation, she began to recover herself, her mind cleared, and she came to realize just how preposterous the whole program of treatment had been. She sought legal remedies for her losses, her long periods of despair, the painful separations, and her sense of guilt for subjecting her children to this kind of abuse.

A long legal battle ensued in the Cook County Circuit Court, and various experts in psychiatry and psychology were brought in to investigate the available records and debate the presumptions justifying the form of treatment that had been used with Burgus. After a series of depositions and meetings with people of various opinions on this case, the insurance companies providing malpractice insurance for Rush Presbyterian Hospital and for its employee Dr. Bennett Braun decided to settle the suit and ultimately paid Burgus $10.6 million.

This large settlement was probably no more than would have been awarded if this woman and her two children had testified in a civil complaint before a jury, which would have heard of the outrageous claims made about them. Evidence that this decision was likely correct came when the State of Illinois, following up on this matter, suspended Braun's medical license. A giant in the MPD movement had been felled.

He certainly did not go quietly. Although he put his treatment programs off limits by citing patient confidentiality, when he was asked specifically about the Croatian cults, he blamed Burgus for it all. "She just spit it out," he said to the *New York Times* reporter covering the case. "All of the cult stuff that she was talking about, I learned from her."

But Braun never denied that he taught medical students and psychiatric residents about satanic cults and that MPD was due to extreme childhood abuse that had been repressed. He never retracted his belief that individuals could repress or dissociate all knowledge of traumatic events, so that a person might have suffered extreme abuse for many years—from early childhood through to adulthood—with no conscious knowledge that such events could have happened or had ever occurred.

Braun didn't deny these ideas—and many therapists did not think he should. To give up on them would have implications far beyond the domain of MPD treatments.

These two paradigm cases of Nadean Cool and Patty Burgus have much in common. In both, each of the accused therapists believed that the human memory is a kind of repository where past events, and particularly trauma experiences, are laid down and permanently stored in a clear and unaltered form. They held that, given this fact, accurate memories can and should be drawn into consciousness in explaining contemporary distress. These foundational assumptions justified the use of hypnosis to "explore" the past life of both of these patients. Both patients, while under hypnosis, told the therapists the stories they expected to find.

These cases demonstrate that hypnosis turns out to "work" the same way that torture "works." The directors "know" what they want the subjects to say, and they "work them over" (with torture or hypnosis) until they hear what they expect to hear.

With hypnosis in these patients, another advantage emerged for those believing in recovered memory. Once these patients began to believe that hypnosis was an appropriate way to "try to remember," each sought out new themes—often themes mentioned and developed during group therapy—and found again that her therapist was a ready listener and encouraged the process.

Because the new themes were naturally seen by all as richer and more explanatory memories, an expansive story line ensued. Before long, everyone in Rush's Department of Psychiatry was imagining life in fifteenth-century Croatia. Under the spell of the hypnotic testimony, what John Mack could believe about alien abduction, Bennett Braun could believe about Satan.

Most of the other cases of malpractice I studied were similar to these. The majority of therapists worked incompetently, much as Dr. Olson did in the Nadean Cool case; they displayed similar mistakes of omission and commission.

Just consider what these doctors didn't do. They failed to take a full psychiatric history from their patients, but instead rested their diagnostic opinions on a list of symptoms that theory taught were "diagnostic of previous child abuse." They launched emotionally evocative cathartic therapies without ever seeking outside informants, such as family members who could describe the patients' characteristics, capacities, and vulnerabilities.

They advanced their treatments but failed to review and reassess their program when, after some months, the patients were more emotionally disturbed and distressed than when they began.

They rationalized these results by interpreting all new symptoms and signs as proof of their original views. The therapists believed emotional outbursts and even occasional suicidal actions were signs that the patients were "working through the implications" of learning what they had repressed. Because the emotions were "appropriate," the treatment was to increase the sedating medications and so keep the patients intoxicated.

The therapists never considered the possibility that the emotional states arising in treatment were the toxic products of their treatment. And, most tellingly, they never sought second opinions from therapists outside the like-minded circle of believers in "recovered memories."

But why were so many therapists committed to practicing in this deeply flawed manner? One likely possibility is that America has more therapists than firemen or mail carriers, and twice as many therapists as dentists or pharmacists, and that there are not enough good educational programs for them. Scant training makes many of them vulnerable to accepting any thera-peutic concept that draws attention, fits with the therapist community's mores of suspicion, and tells them what to do when a "client" knocks on the door. Recovered memory therapy could be taken off the rack—ready-made, as it were—presented in handbooks like *The Courage to Heal*. Given their numbers, their inadequate training, their lack of a critical sense, and the growing competition among them for patients, why should anyone be surprised by what they did and the damage they caused?

But Dr. Braun was not one of these untrained therapists. He was in academic psychiatry, and his ideas had received support—and still do—in centers of education in the country.

Indeed, his practice was sustained by a "movement" within the psychiatric profession—a movement related to the psychoanalytic movement. All this made it possible for him to claim that his treatment met standards and to blame the patient for the outcome.

Perhaps the clearest way to appreciate this movement and what protects these practitioners from punishment is to see Manneristic Freudians as Freudian "heretics." They remain committed to Freudian ideas of the unconscious, particularly its importance as the site of early memories of sexual and emotional conflicts. They agree with orthodox Freudians about how these conflicts generate fantasies, dreams, and mental problems, and how the conflicts work their way into therapies where "transference and resistance" are in play. Their heresy resides in their belief that *actual* sexual abuse rather than conflicted sexual *desire* is at the heart of the problem.

Thus Dr. Braun, like all heretics, held to the fundamentals but applied them in the service of the new claim. Demonstrating how his case went wrong would not undermine belief in "recovered memories," because classic, standard, everyday Freudian psychology supports the ideas of memory and repression on which that belief rests. As long as most psychiatrists continue to think that Freud was correct when he said "in mental life nothing which has once been formed can perish,"[2] then the practices and ideas tied to "recovered memories" will persist no matter how many shocking cases like that of Patty Burgus come along.

Something much more radical than malpractice judgments will be needed. And this is how I've come to see the problem after all my experiences in court.

Just as Galileo and Descartes turned around the astronomical cosmology of their day (and so overthrew the metaphysical basis of the Middle Ages that supported witch trials), only a new psychology—essentially a new "cosmology of the mind"—will eliminate practices that support memory recovery therapies.

Even more specifically: to end support for what Richard Ofshe dubbed the "robust repression" behind MPD and "recovered memories," one must offer an approach to the mind and memory that does away even with the concept of "ordinary repression" and its role in mental life. This means repudiating a system of thought rather than pointing out a "simple mistake." The contemporary psychological investigators of memory, such as Elizabeth Loftus, Daniel Schacter, Larry Squire, and Richard McNally, who trace their methods to those great American psychological Galileos,

William James and Karl Lashley, must draw clinical psychiatrists away from "searching memory" with hypnosis and other suggestive means.

But if the psychological cosmology of psychoanalysis persists, the real lessons of the Cool and Braun cases will never be learned. Those unwilling or unprepared to question central Freudian psychology can deal with the Nadean Cool and Patty Burgus treatments in two ways, and neither of these positions is radical enough to put an end to the intellectual belief in recovered memories.

One way is to dismiss these cases as merely examples of the incompetent application of a correct set of assumptions. There's plenty of incompetence to go around, and this approach is the least demanding position to assume.

Another way is to take on a scholastic skepticism and propose that some middle ground exists between the energetic believers in recovered memory ("who will sometimes be right") and the energetic disbelievers ("who also will sometimes be right"). This, as I mentioned earlier, is an effort in *political* compromise, rather than a *scientific* position. It gains support among those who, looking for an easy solution, do the least to confirm any opinion—left, right, or center—with data.

As H. R. Trevor-Roper points out in his classic essay on the European witch craze of the sixteenth and seventeenth centuries,[3] this empirically ambiguous posture was precisely the approach taken by Montaigne, the most influential pundit of his time. It allowed him to seem wise and yet left the witch craze exactly where he found it, and with innocents still being hunted and killed.

The posture of scholastic skepticism and political compromise is embedded in the *DSM* classification of dissociative identity disorder (as might be expected, given that, as I'll describe in a later chapter, the authors of *DSM-III* had to make "deals" to get the manual accepted). It describes what patients with dissociative identity disorder look like but ignores whether these appearances depend on a valid mechanism of memory or represent a behavioral artifact built on psychological assumptions. As a result, *DSM* leaves the issues of recovered memory cases right where it found them. And not surprisingly, the thinking behind these cases is being employed once again to confuse the public about Vietnam veterans, another topic I shall discuss in a later chapter.

But what will happen with the issue of MPD and recovered memories? The problem of the many incompetent therapists will not change as long as there are people ready to go to therapists on their own, without a competent psychiatric evaluation and prescription, accepting therapy as a kind of "tonic." But heavy fines and malpractice suits can help suppress enthusiasm for developing "personalities" in patients and claiming memories were "recovered."

The Mannerists persist—encouraged by *DSM*—but have become moving targets. They remain hard to pin down on case management and are changing their terminology and claiming to have progressed. The old MPD units are being renamed "trauma treatment" or "trauma disorder programs." Most important to the Mannerists is their hope of preserving the concept of MPD as a real disorder by renaming it dissociative identity disorder.

A nice example is the way a star Mannerist, Dr. David Spiegel, has worked to erase the idea of "multiple personalities" by saying that MPD patients do not have more than one personality but actually have "less than one." By this odd turn of phrase, he means that the minds of these patients have been "shattered" by trauma and that the "alters" are "fragments" of mind.

This idea sounds very wise, but it still depends on a view of memory that presumes it can be divided up and split off—such that memories are accessible to some parts of consciousness and inaccessible to other parts. It continues to suppose that feelings and memories are buried in some vaults where they remain intact, even if accessible only by one of those "fragments" that were once called "alters." *Nothing* in the contemporary science of human memory supports this idea. Spiegel's concept—more than one but less than one—is a device for sustaining a clinical posture, and a rather incoherent one when closely inspected.

Finally, as I spent time with injured patients discussing what had happened to them, I saw them struggling for a sense of purpose. They had, with help, come to retract their accusations against their families and realize what they had done to injure themselves and bring shame to all.

But many found themselves back where they started, with the same lack of direction in life that sent them to a therapist in the first place. They had difficulty imagining what to do next. They were set up for relapse.

Considerable follow-up care was needed by them. Those who found coherent therapies of the kind I'll describe later in this book did well. Those who were abandoned to their own devices had difficulty in finding a full recovery. They remained victims of the continuing battles over psychiatric practice.

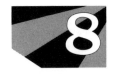

Getting to Know Patients

The clearest perception that I gathered from these battles over multiple personality and recovered memories was that, time and again, these psychiatrists and therapists just did not know their patients. They were blinded by theory and saw them in an overly simple way—always as "victims."

Because these therapists either did not concede or failed to realize that identical mental symptoms can emerge from very different provocations, they did not try to differentiate their patients' conditions, nor did they use comprehensive methods to illuminate what their patients actually faced. Rather, they drew conclusions on the basis of a few symptoms, they delivered those conclusions and their implications to the patients without reflection, they encouraged violent emotional reactions, and they never revised their opinions when the patients did poorly.

This means that psychiatrists who are called to help patients previously treated for MPD or given false memories have to "go back to basics" in caring for them. Just what these are, why they apply to cases of this sort, and how they encourage proper practices make the basics of great interest in themselves.

Serious and competent psychiatrists have long been aware that they can muddle up clinical problems if they approach their patients without a sound and comprehensive system for gathering pertinent information. In his 1943 classic, *Outlines for Psychiatric Examinations*, Nolan D. C. Lewis noted:

> Owing to the variety and complexity of the situations dealt with in the investigation of life histories and the difficulties encountered in the examination of many types of mental disorder, the student or physician who approaches a case without a definite plan in mind is certain to overlook important facts or permit the patient to lead too much in the examination, often with the result that the time is not spent to the best advantage or that he is misled into drawing false conclusions.[1]

Adolf Meyer, who was the prominent American teacher of psychiatry in the first half of the twentieth century, held that all psychological symptoms and disorders in one way or another are to be seen as emerging from the life as lived. Although we see things somewhat differently today, given that we recognize how some diseases of mind such as schizophrenia and bipolar disorder disrupt the course of mental life rather than "emerge" from it, we do continue to hold that symptoms are always shaped by personality and life experience. Hence we teach the need for a biographical assessment of every patient. Not only does this assessment help place symptoms into context, but it specifically draws attention to the way a patient dealt with the milestones of life that all of us must meet and manage.

Distinctive features of personality—strengths, weaknesses, habitual responses, virtues, and vices—are revealed by the characteristic ways in which a person has coped with the issues of growth and development, education, employment, sex and marital life, and social and legal responsibilities. In similar ways, how medical, surgical, or psychological disruptions were met and overcome provide crucial knowledge about the person and what might be expected from him or her when new challenges arise.

Because accuracy in a biographical history is crucial, psychiatrists must seek to confirm and add further to the biographical facts by meeting with those other people ("external informants" or "independent observers") who have long known the patient and often have crucial information about the onset of the problem that brought the person to seek treatment.

The review of the patient with a close relative was always a requirement in psychiatry before the emergence of the Freudian School of Suspicion. And this is again reflected in the Lewis manual where he clearly states, "The practice should be to try always to get the anamnesis [i.e., history] from relatives or friends, as in many instances one cannot depend on the patient for the previous history as is usually done in general medical cases."[2]

Knowledge of the biographical background of the patient helps in identifying how the present symptoms emerged. Were they new and unexpected, or were they a repetition of previous problems now more intense and more prolonged? Here psychiatrists consider such matters as the acute or chronic nature of the symptoms, what form they initially took, what other symptoms accompanied them, and whether they changed in character, intensity, or duration over time.

Psychiatrists must learn what previous treatments, if any, were sought and given, and whether these treatments relieved or worsened the patient's condition. Psychiatric interviews customarily close with an examination of the states of mind presented by the patients: how they look, how they speak, what seems to be preoccupying them the most, and in particular how they respond to the process of being questioned and cross-questioned about their past history and their present condition.

This process of assessment can take several hours and frequently requires separate sessions over several days to complete. Extra time—separate from the patient—is needed as the doctor seeks remote external informants to describe the patient's personality, habitual responses, and sequences of development and engagement with daily life.

But taking a history from a patient who comes into the office with MPD and recovered memories often is particularly awkward. While most previously treated patients have ideas about their problem, these patients are especially difficult to win round to a new beginning. Often they are not interested in reviewing their lives with yet another psychiatrist. They "know" that their depressions, anxieties, eating disorders, or interpersonal problems are the products of childhood or adolescent sexual abuse now remembered years after the events. And they expect the psychiatrist to agree.

In the early 1990s, I saw many such patients. They came with something specific in mind—such as getting my support in a parental or legal encounter—and quickly revealed that intention when early in their visit they asked something like, "Do you believe in multiple personalities?" or "Do you believe in repressed memories?" How I answered determined what followed, including whether they would continue the consultation.

I learned that if I registered the slightest doubt about MPD or recovered memories, the meeting would quickly end—often unpleasantly. Several patients shouted insults at me and bolted from the office.

Because I could neither assess nor help a patient who would not stay, I learned to respond to these questions by pointing out what was quite true—that no one has an unlimited experience and that I was still learning from patients about what exists and what might trouble them. I tried to promote the idea that we should give each other some time to think through the situation together.

Perhaps, I now say to a patient, once I go over her story—the vast majority of these patients are women—I can suggest something about how to proceed that might improve on her present plans or on the treatments she has been receiving. This maneuver usually, but not always, leads to a wary truce in which opinions and decisions are held at bay so as to permit at least the preliminary steps in a clinical evaluation to proceed.

As my first step, I explain what's involved in a psychiatric assessment that might lead to treatment. I do this even though the patients usually have seen some mental health worker before. I want to make clear what the patient and I should expect from each other if we proceed. A useful term for this exercise within the psychiatric assessment process is "role induction."

This step surprises many patients. Although they had been in one or another kind of therapy, no one had spelled out what it entails, what can be expected, and what responsibilities the doctor and patient must carry for good outcomes to emerge. Their previous therapists simply began asking about their symptoms and then told them "what the symptoms said."

Some patients were suspicious of this first action of mine. But I could truthfully explain that good psychotherapists often repeat the role induction process several times when working with patients because of the benefits it brings.

The first thing I say during this process is that psychiatric evaluations and treatments are not familiar experiences to most people and that many have false ideas about them. Psychiatrists who clarify their purposes and their methods to patients seem to do better than those who don't. I then explain that psychiatric evaluations, resting on dialogue between doctor and patient, depend on the patient's trust and cooperation. Role induction offers patients early in the encounter the opportunity to engage in "give and take" or "feedback" in which the psychiatrist can answer questions, relieve anxiety, dispel any mystery or false impressions, and encourage a willingness to proceed. During role induction, doctors can explain and patients can ask about the process of evaluation or therapy, what if any dangers may come with it, and what is ultimately involved.

Through the role induction process, I hope to move to the diagnostic interview itself, in which I strive to gain a full picture of the patient's history. My aim is to make sense both of what originally brought the patient to psychiatric attention and what provoked the idea of MPD and "memories." As I mentioned earlier, however, the patient has usually come with her own "story"—an account of sexual abuse, dissociation, or multiple personalities—and, as Lewis warned, may strive to lead the examination.

A good example is a young woman who came to my office along with her married sister, whom she had told she "remembered" how their father had sexually abused her at puberty. Until recently, the young woman had had an excellent and friendly relationship with her father, who had been quite indulgent with her. Since she left home for college, some ten years earlier, she had stayed in touch, writing and sending many affectionate cards to both her parents and returning home on frequent friendly visits.

Her major problem had been finding a stable intimate relationship that might lead to the marriage and family life she hoped for—hardly an uncommon issue for young people. She had had boyfriends, but they had been rather "rough" types, and she had cohabited for a time with a drug addict. Recently she had been depressed and preoccupied with the sense that her life was not "making progress." She consulted with a therapist, who promptly told her that her difficulties with men were the result of her being a "sex abuse victim" and that therapy would involve "trying to remember" her injuries.

She had no memory at all of any sexual abuse in her life, but was willing to devote several sessions to reviewing her childhood with the therapist. They finally concluded that her father had indeed been overly preoccupied with her development at puberty and must have abused her, and although the patient couldn't quite remember the details of the sexual abuse, she did remember times when she felt angry with her father. She and the therapist agreed that these were probably remnant feelings following a sexual assault which she had undergone but promptly "repressed."

In the following weeks, she had dreams that she thought confirmed her fears. The problem was that neither her moods nor her confidence improved. Rather, she became more and more upset and preoccupied by her worries over past abuse. For this reason, she called her sister in Baltimore to see if she had also been abused. Her sister persuaded her to see me. And here she was.

She quickly made it clear, though, that she had not come looking for my help in treatment. She had come to see me so that I would convince her sister that she was a "victim" of their father—a story that made "sense" of her problems in life. She came looking for someone to confirm the story and to deal with problems that had become too difficult for her. A conflict of stories as much as a conflict of diagnoses produces quite a clinical challenge.

Before I could review her life history and the onset of these beliefs about her father, I had to deal with the emotional state she presented and her demands for my support. "Don't you agree that I've the symptoms of someone sexually abused?" she asked. I could only reply that certainly her feelings were understandable, given her beliefs, but that maybe, if we turned to look at what else could explain the problems for which she had originally sought therapy, we might turn up something helpful for planning a future. "Let's try to look ahead for awhile rather than forever concentrating on the past," I suggested.

Because she came with her sister, I had the opportunity to go over just what her past life was like, at least as seen from the perspective of someone who knew her well and cared about her. The sister described just how emotionally volatile the patient had always been. She described her as lively, emotionally responsive, and affectionate, but easily irritated sometimes by trifles and prone to hold grudges. She was the more adventurous of their family and sometimes did take up with new fads and wilder types of friends. She was stubborn and would hold out for her own way when arguing with her family. The sister worried that now she would hold to her opinions about the abuse and separate from all of them, including her if she didn't agree with the charges against their father.

My efforts turned to winning the patient around to a treatment program that would not continue along the same path that she had been following. I mentioned that she was so distressed that her emotions were now in the way. I recommended that she cease seeing her present therapist ("at least for a time") and that she work with a female psychiatrist who would be both sympathetic and open to her views but who would concentrate on helping her work out what stood in her way now rather than digging in the past. I thought that would relieve some of her present distress and that we'd see what turned up after a few weeks or months of such treatment.

I proposed that plan because of what I thought the evidence indicated. I thought the patient had been through a stressful period, worrying about her future and particularly about her prospects for marriage after an awkward breakup with a boyfriend. Her discouragement and demoralization at that time needed to be treated with some reassurance and reminders of the assets she already possessed. More effort should be placed on guiding her ways of thinking about her future and how she made decisions related to romantic partners.

Instead, she had been launched into a therapy of "try to remember" and experienced the expected outcome of resentment and alienation. As I'll describe below, I thought the probability of abuse here was minimal, although there were reasons for believing that the father did mishandle the delicate matters of puberty in this emotionally high-strung woman. There would need to be a long "time-out period" to permit her feelings to quiet down—and this could occur only if these feelings were not being reawakened with every therapy session.

And so it worked out. After a two-year period of separation from her father, the patient, who did find a suitable husband, agreed that "perhaps I exaggerated the problem with Dad" and reconciled with him.

A patient such as this one shows how a psychiatrist can diagnostically reassess the initiating problems that launched a patient into false beliefs and family crisis. Also, this patient had never been taught that psychotherapy can work by helping patients look forward rather than backward, and that we all might "give it a trial" without any confrontation over her beliefs. A treatment plan focusing on how she thought about herself and her boyfriends turned out to work well for her.

But what about patients who bring with them a diagnosis of MPD (or DID, as many might call the same condition today)? The "back-to-basics" clinician would, even before launching a role induction, have some opinion about the problem and the issues it raises. These issues are: What is the nature of MPD? What does it represent? How is it like or different from other psychiatric conditions? and How might the answers to such questions promote rational treatment? Following are my answers.

First, MPD is not a natural condition produced in a natural way by the mind faced with a life event. Thus it is not in the class of species-specific stereotypic mental responses, such as the emotional state of grief that follows losing someone precious or the anxious states of mind that accompany and follow traumatic experiences.

MPD certainly does not belong in the class of conditions produced by some disruption of the brain mechanisms responsible for memory, such as seen in patients who have suffered a concussive injury like a "knockout punch" or have received electroconvulsive treatment (ECT) for depression. These traumas both affect the memory of events that happened shortly before the blow (retrograde amnesia) and for a time eliminate the capacity to form new memories about the events that follow it (anterograde amnesia).

Rather than any of these kinds of clinical problems, MPD is by nature a behavior taken up by the patient in order to meet the expectations of, win the support of, or otherwise satisfy other people who carry power to affect the future. These include doctors who can wield the benefits of the medical system, relatives who can provide domestic and financial resources, or jurists who can exert civil sanctions and criminal punishments.

MPD falls into the class of behaviors that include those mimicking medical illnesses, such as pseudo-seizures or factitious palsies; those deriving from social expectations, such as the trances seen in the Charcot clinic; and those emerging during local panics, such as the "fits" of the girls in the Salem witch trials (I will go into more detail about these famous cases in Chapter 10).

Like all these other examples, the behavior of MPD patients is expressed in ways that others construe and interpret as evidence of a hidden injury. MPD is thus a behavior made legitimate by and maintained through the social interactions it evokes with significant others. It is a socially constructed pattern of behavior.

Again, to make sense of it and bring it under control, the psychiatrist must know both the patient and the situation rewarding the behavior. Then the psychiatrist can manage the problem and prove its social nature by changing the rewards and watching the behavior disappear. And this is what many in my profession have learned to do when MPD patients come to us.

As a first step, we separate the patient from any therapist who is seeing her, encouraging her memories, or "eliciting" her "alter" personalities. This requires some negotiation, and often the best way to accomplish it is to persuade the patient to enter the hospital for a week and to direct treatment toward some specific and pressing symptom—her depression, her anorexia, or her angry outbursts. Such an approach interrupts the sustaining and provoking attention that comes from talking about "alters."

In the role induction, the patient should be told that the treatment of these "simpler" issues—again, the depression, anorexia, or what have you-will take place without efforts to review the past. The staff, the patient must be told, will attend solely to matters in the here and now in her life.

If the patient displays any of the "dissociative" phenomena, such as multiple personalities, fugues, or periods of amnesia, these behaviors are ignored by the staff. And if the patient objects, she is coaxed back on track by being told that these "dissociative episodes" are transient remnants of her prior illness and now that recovery is under way, she shouldn't worry about them.

Again, all this is done without any reprise of the old story and reference to her claims of abuse. Occasionally the patient will make threats of doing herself harm or leaving our care, but again attention directed at the anorexia or depression and how these symptoms remain as great burdens to her usually brings her around.

The patient may try to win some nurses or other patients over to her "story" and in that way split up the team into those "supporting" and those "denying" the patient's story. We overcome this effort by having regular team conferences, with doctors, nurses, social workers, and occupational therapists all together listening to just how incapacitated the patient has become by the story she believes.

When asked by allies of the patient as to the truth or falseness of the story, the doctors or nurses should reply quite honestly: "It's too early to say. And in a sense it's too tough for us to manage. Let's deal with what's in front of us and see what happens."

What surprises many people is that multiple personalities tend to fall away quickly when ignored. Usually on our anorexia nervosa floor, patients who entered with MPD cease discussing their alters within a few days and often report that after a week or two of recovering their body weight and attending group therapy tied to their eating disorder, the ideas and preoccupations with their "alters" gradually vanished from their thinking.

If patients arrive with MPD and it falls away with neglect, then sometimes the issue of remembered sexual abuse disappears along with it. But not always. Their therapists may well have been telling them something similar to what the therapists told Donna Smith: "If you have not been telling the truth about what you remembered, then you're much sicker than we thought."

Psychiatrists should begin by acknowledging that they cannot prejudge the matter. Even though most of the patients who have been treated with various forms of recovered memory therapy present very dubious evidence for their beliefs—and numbers of them have recanted their original positions—nothing available at the start of an inquiry permits anyone to assume that the patient is mistaken.

Despite a wealth of evidence that shocking experiences such as sexual assaults are virtually impossible to forget, the theory of "dissociation" has put a new burden on psychiatrists to show that they have considered the possibility that a memory can be completely forgotten and then brought to mind in therapy. Thus psychiatrists have a responsibility to decide whether the belief as presented by the patient at hand is probable or improbable.

To meet this responsibility—and to challenge the recovered memory therapists to do the same—we at Hopkins have employed a method used by epidemiologists and public health workers. It is called a "2 × 2," or "four-fold," table. With it we can see the problem clearly, as it ties together the issues of abuse experiences and memories of abuse in a way that defines the diagnostic problem and what is needed to solve it.

The table relies on the fact that we can separate the human population into those who have been abused and those who have not. This division forms the two vertical columns of the table. The table also uses the fact that we can separate everyone into those who think they were abused (who harbor a memory of an abuse event) and those who don't think they were abused (who harbor no memory of an abuse event). This second division of the population forms the two crossing horizontal rows of the table. The intersection of columns and rows produces four cells, in which everyone has a place.

TRUTH

	Abused	Not Abused
Memory	HIT	FALSE ALARM
No Memory	FORGOTTEN	FREE

As with any 2 × 2 table, there are people in each of the four cells. There are those who have been abused and remember the abuse (Hits). There are people who have been abused and do not remember it. They may not have recognized the event as a form of sexual abuse when it happened, the event may have happened when they were too young to remember, or they may have forgotten the event in the same way other events fade in memory. Whatever the explanation, these people fall into the Forgotten cell. There are, fortunately, many people who have never been abused and have no memories of abuse (Free). Finally, we know that some people have memories of abuse and never were abused (False Alarms). Among the False Alarms are people who make extraordinary claims, including those who believe they were carried off by aliens and abused in a spacecraft.

This table makes clear what psychiatrists face when a patient comes in saying that she has "recovered" a memory of abuse. The psychiatrist must decide what column the patient "ascended" when she moved from "No Memory" to "Memory." The patient would present herself in the same way whether she ascended the "Abused" column (from Forgotten to Hit) or the "Not Abused" column (from Free to False Alarm). She would claim to have "recovered" a memory in either case.

Psychiatrists faced with a patient saying she has "recovered" a memory must decide which column the patient ascended, because on that decision much will depend—the therapy to be followed, the reports issued, the future relationships of families. In making that decision psychiatrists must turn to the actual history of the patient's "remembering."

Several aspects of that history illuminate the issue diagnostically: (1) the content of the memory, (2) the genesis of the memory, (3) any confirmation of the memory, and (4) the settings of the memory recovery.

Thus the content of the memory will be important to consider. If the patient says that the abuse happened when she was of school age, that the abuser was well known to her, that the abuse was a private affair and produced trouble for her at the time, and that she has wondered ever since whether to bring forth her complaints or simply "forget" about them, then diagnosticians should feel confident that they're dealing with someone reporting an actual event and begin to deal with the consequences.

How different this content of memory is from that of a patient who says she was abused when she was an infant during diaper changes, or that the abuse took place as an aspect of a satanic ritual in which her family and neighbors all were taking part, and that despite many physical injuries and terrible experiences, this abuse never interfered with her well-witnessed capacity to attend school, have happy friendships, and move forward in her physical and emotional development. With this story some doubts are surely justified, and inquiry into how the memory was generated naturally follows.

Considering the genesis of the memory is useful. If the patient says that she has actually always known of the abuse but had either minimized its importance or put it out of her mind until recently, when she began to worry about matters of personal integrity and her future well-being, diagnosticians would surely feel more confident that they were dealing with someone who has remembered an actual event. They would contrast this story with one in which the patient reports that she developed her memory when she was in therapy with a therapist who drew her attention to the possibility of abuse right from the start and used hypnotic inductions and repetitive trances to "recover" the memory, that the memory only slowly emerged from the mists of confusion and concern provoked in the therapeutic process, and that she was prompted to remember by reading books like *The Courage to Heal*, along with receiving encouragement from other members of a group of "incest survivors" who claimed her depressive or anxious symptoms "typified" those of the sexually abused.

As for the confirmation of the memory: If the patient brings witnesses or confessions from the perpetrator about the abuse and demonstrates just how disrupted her life was for some time during the period of abuse, again diagnosticians would feel more confident that they're dealing with someone who is reporting a memory of an actual event than if the patient reports that "because of her repression" she remained a perfectly successful schoolgirl and a happy-seeming child to her parents even though she had been impregnated, had had several abortions, and was repeatedly abused without either of her parents knowing about those events or witnessing the injuries when she was being bathed or dressed.

The settings in which the memory was recovered also influence one's decision. If the patient had many previous psychiatric consultations for depression, anxiety, and anorexia and regularly reported her abuse history, certainly a psychiatrist would have more confidence in the memory's validity than in that of a claim that emerged only when clinicians used hypnosis and suggestion to evoke and sustain a new belief about the patient's past.

For myself, after these reflections and examinations, I'm usually in a position to offer a reasonably confident opinion as to why I think the patient, upon "recovering" a memory, ascended one or the other column and exemplifies a Hit or a False Alarm. For example, with the young woman whose sister brought her to see me, I noted that her memories were generated under therapeutic pressure, they were "recovered" with some difficulty, and a "search" was required to fix on her father. They were not confirmed by any other evidence and flew in the face of the past warm feelings the patient had shown for her father. I concluded that she had ascended from Free to a False Alarm. That she ultimately retracted her memory seemed to confirm my view.

I certainly do not believe I'm always correct in my decision, or that anyone who disagrees must be wrong. I continue to seek and accept evidence for the contrary opinion. But I do know that if others interested in and concerned for patients who have been sexually mistreated approached the diagnostic problem more systematically, then much of the confusion generated by the Manneristic Freudians with their "recovered memory" claims would disappear.

Malpractice claims also would stop, because many of the malpractice claims rest upon the fact that the hospital records show only the effort to confirm a preconception rather than any good faith enterprise, such as that demanded by the 2 × 2 table. With such records, many judges and juries conclude that the therapists were not thinking about their diagnostic responsibility. And when the patient retracts and complains about mistreatment, the sense that the therapist was promoting a belief rather than acting dispassionately in the patient's interest will advance. As doctors are taught right from the start of their clinical work, neglect of an obvious responsibility leads to malpractice claims far more often than does an honest error.

Conclusion: Know the patient. On that all else depends.

And yet many therapists have raised objections to these principles of assessment and treatment. Some assume that the approach underestimates the diagnostic significance of "dissociation" and the display of multiple "alters" and how this behavior *in itself* points to a trauma history. "What else could it be?" one of the MPD experts asked me. Others claim that clinicians know things from their long experience and that I am missing—perhaps "willfully" missing—deeper and more significant matters of importance in psychiatric disorders that depend on recovering memories.

My onetime opponent at the *Quattrocchi* hearing, Dr. Paul Applebaum, who regularly defended treatments based on recovered memories, once dismissed critics like me who had pointed out the injuries suffered by a gifted Harvard medical student who had undergone such treatments by saying that psychotherapy is "not the same as making Toll House cookies."

Indeed it is not. Neither is it like pulling a rabbit out of a hat: The ways of practicing psychiatry and psychotherapy should be coherent and fully transparent to any interested observer. If those who practice in these disciplines draw a curtain of mystery over their methods, approaches, aims, and outcomes, then not only are they doing their patients and the public a great disservice, but they and their associates will often lose their way and come to grief—as happened to the practitioners of "recovered memory" therapy I've been describing here.

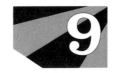

Making Sense of
DSM

W hen I propose that multiple personality disorder is a behavioral artifact rather than a natural mental disorder, the most critical question I encounter is, "Well, it's listed in *DSM*, is it not?" I've learned that more than a probing interest may prompt this remark. The inquirer often intends to suggest that if psychiatry's mainstream manual lists the condition, then not only must it exist as a natural condition—along with its connotations about hidden trauma, memory repression, "alters," and the like—but, more to the point, "rational" psychiatrists must see these matters as settled.

I reply—in the hope that the question comes in good faith—by noting that we all might reflect on what to conclude about any of the disorders listed in *DSM-III* and *-IV* (which I will refer to jointly as *DSM-III/IV*).[1] For I believe that in order to respond to the question "If it's in the *DSM*, isn't it real?" one must delve into how medical and surgical diagnostic classifications work and just how *DSM-III/IV* differs from them.

Distinctions crucial to the question at hand rest on this difference, and those who appreciate that difference understand why an entry in *DSM* does not certify a diagnostic entity as "real." Also, they will promptly grasp how the strange set of ideas culminating in MPD could wade into the mainstream of American psychiatry and cause such mischief.

Medicine and surgery have long used a "systematic" classification represented now by the tenth edition of the *International Classification of Disease* (*ICD-10*). Here clinical disorders are differentiated first by what caused them—pathologic processes such as infections, malignancies, faulty genes, or traumatic injuries—and second by how these causal processes injure the functional "machinery" of the organs they attack, such as the heart, the lungs, or the brain.

Medical classifications thus grasp—through cause and mechanism—what doctors believe to be the nature of each medical condition and the source of its symptoms (i.e., "This patient's condition belongs among the infectious disorders of the lung—the pneumonias—hence the patient's breathlessness, cough, and fever"). The classification also indicates how critical students can confirm or refute a diagnosis by searching out its implications—such as by showing with X-rays the clouding of the lung in pneumonia or by demonstrating the pneumococcal bacteria in the patient's sputum.

ICD-10 describes the common symptoms of each disorder to identify how the condition ordinarily presents itself. But it also stipulates how similar symptoms can arise from very different conditions and so emphasizes that symptoms don't tell the whole story.

This approach to classification by cause and mechanism was not always used in medicine. Until late in the nineteenth century, patients' disorders were classified according to their physical expressions (epilepsy and dropsy, for example) or according to their symptoms. A favored method was classifying patients by describing the repetitive fever courses they followed.

As late as 1868, Carl Wunderlich, a German physician, could publish *The Variation of the Body Heat in Illnesses,* a massive treatise in which he classified a large group of illnesses according to their characteristic fever curves— that is, the fever patterns the patients displayed over time. This book made doctors diagnostically consistent (or "reliable") with febrile patients (that is, they agreed with one another in the diagnoses they assigned to the patients), but it failed miserably in identifying the nature of the clinical disorders, because many different medical conditions produce identical fever patterns. Wunderlich had offered a reliable approach to medical diagnosis, but not one from which rational treatments or coherent predictions could be drawn.

Less than fifteen years later, Robert Koch, the physician and bacteriologist, provided the first classification of febrile illnesses based on the infectious agents that caused them. His method of classifying illnesses led directly to discovering ways of treating and preventing the diseases. It promptly supplanted the Wunderlich approach.

Medicine has continued in the way pioneered by Koch: classify disorders according to presumed causes—even when the cause is complicated and untreatable—because this way of classifying will gradually approach a description of nature itself. Other causes for illness besides infection will come to be discovered, rational treatments will be discerned, and the ways to prove that the conditions identified are real products of nature will become clear to everyone.

This way of classifying medical disorders brought two other valuable assets. First, it provided a means of assuring doctors that when they made a diagnosis—confirmed both by the characteristics of the patient and the tests performed—other doctors could reach the same diagnostic conclusion. Outcomes could be compared and treatment findings "replicated" in other clinics and other patients because doctors could be sure they were studying similar conditions.

Second, this classification based on causes and mechanisms would encourage research into how causes could be interrupted or their effects ameliorated. In this way, a fully rational scientific medicine expands and the physicians themselves become more and more effective.

This, in brief, has been the history of classification and practice in medicine and surgery for the past 140 years. The standard clinical method of inductive reasoning emerged from combining this way of defining medical disorders by cause and mechanism with methods of examining patients—their histories, physical states, and laboratory results—for evidence. More causes for medical and surgical disorders were discovered, and more effective treatments emerged.

Just as important, the public gained confidence in the reality of the conditions the doctors identify and treat. Most people now expect their doctors to explain the disorders they suffer and the treatments they must undergo in ways they can understand using concepts derived from the study of nature.

This public confidence in the reality of medical disorders probably led to the belief that listing MPD in *DSM* must mean that MPD is just as "real." But the contemporary psychiatric classificatory manual (*DSM*) is entirely different from the medical manual. It is not "systematic" but uses a method more like that of old Wunderlich, being a diagnostic system based on symptom patterns rather than causes. And this affects how one must think about any condition it lists.

To appreciate these implications, one must understand two aspects of *DSM-III/IV*. First, its history: how and why it was devised by the leaders of the discipline. Second, its method: what it represents as a diagnostic tool and what benefits and problems it brings.

First, its history: In the late 1970s the leaders of psychiatry—needing a new classification system for the late twentieth century for reasons I'll soon explain—were unable to organize mental disorders systematically by their causes and mechanisms because not only were many unknown, but the issues of causation had provoked furious disputes in the field. Some psychiatrists wished to emphasize dysfunctions of the brain as the cause of psychiatric disorders, while others were holding fast to Freudian causal theories.

In default, psychiatry's leaders turned to symptom patterns because, whether psychiatrists thought unconscious conflicts or biological mechanisms produced mental disorders, they could at least come to agree about the symptoms patients displayed. The prime mover in this process was Dr. Robert Spitzer of Columbia University, who had the remarkable talent of persuading psychiatrists to accept this compromise by arguing that—in the long run—a classification based on causes and nature would emerge from it.

Fundamentally, Dr. Spitzer and his associates advancing *DSM-III* explained that before psychiatrists could even hope to build a systematic classification based on the causes of mental illnesses (a "valid" conception of their natures), they needed to have a manual for identifying and distinguishing one condition from another—a way of becoming "reliable" in their diagnoses. This would enable psychiatric investigators to study disorders individually, "replicate" findings from clinic to clinic, and eventually resolve the disputes over the nature of these conditions.

To achieve diagnostic agreement ("reliability"), the authors of *DSM-III* offered as diagnostic criteria (or "keys" to the diagnostic decisions) the symptoms that "experts" in each disorder claimed to be characteristic of it. The *DSM-III* authors in seeking diagnostic reliability were willing to put aside *everything else* that might matter about a mental disorder—its cause, its generative mechanisms, its provocation, its links to other disorders, and *any* sense of its nature—for the sake of identifiable features that "experts" claimed they used when diagnosing the condition.

Spitzer's team combined a political aim with a classificatory method. They wanted to get American psychiatrists to agree on these "defining" symptoms and then use them in their practice and research. They thought all psychiatrists would then draw closer together as they become consistent in their diagnostic practices. A patient identified as an example of major depression in Baltimore would be so identified if he or she was seen in San Francisco or New Orleans.

They saw no other way forward given the disputatious nature of the discipline. Without reliability in diagnosis—a way of agreeing about what condition one was seeing—psychiatrists would be unable to cooperate in the kind of practice and research that would eventually bridge their differences by revealing the nature of mental disorders.

Research results must be confirmed (i.e., "replicated" by others) before they are to be believed and ultimately put to use. If investigators cannot agree about whether they are studying the same condition, then any claimed discovery—whether that discovery is of a gene causing the disorder or a medication alleviating it—will remain unverified because the next investigator cannot be certain what patients to work with in replicating the finding. Investigators hoping to advance the discipline will remain isolated from one another and unable to affect how psychiatrists think or practice.

To summarize the history: the authors of *DSM-III* believed that in the absence of diagnostic reliability, no way of agreeing on causes of mental disorders would emerge. The best they could do in 1980 was to forge a classification based on symptoms and defer building a classification on causes until the research was done. A systematic, valid classificatory system—one based on a grasp of the nature of mental disorders—they thought would have to wait for another day.

And now turning to method: In deferring to "experts" for their diagnostic criteria, the authors of *DSM-III* had to put their trust in two things: first, that the "experts" really did know the symptomatic identifying features of a disorder, and second, that the disorder the "experts" described really did exist as they believed.

Some of this trust was misplaced. Certain disorders—one of them being MPD—are artifacts constructed by enterprising advocates, who pressed the authors of *DSM-III* to accept them as real. How they could succeed rested on an essential aspect of *DSM* as a classification system.

By organizing disorders according to their symptomatic "appearances," the authors of *DSM-III/IV* (whether they realized it or not) produced a field guide indistinguishable in attributes from field guides used by naturalists.

Field guides permit students of trees, wildflowers, or birds to identify the objects of their interest by pointing out distinctions in their appearance. Roger Tory Peterson's *Field Guide to the Birds* found fame as "the birder's bible" not because it defines the birds or organizes them into rough classes—putting the ducks with the ducks and the warblers with the warblers—but because, with the help of "experts," Peterson highlighted those easily spotted "field marks" of bodily shape, plumage, color, and voice that most clearly distinguish birds from one another "on the fly." From his field guide we learn that the European Starling is the only black bird with a yellow bill in North America—an interesting fact, but one that tells us little about the bird of the sort to satisfy an ornithologist's aim of explaining its nature, history, and proliferation on our continent.

The field guide method for identifying different types of plants or animals brings "diagnostic" reliability to the amateur naturalist. It serves such efforts as census-taking and sample-collecting. In particular, its "diagnostic" reliability helps most when knowledge of these objects is limited or primitive, in that it reassures those seeking new knowledge that they are studying an object that others have identified.

Yet even as a method of identification, field guides have several serious weaknesses. They say nothing about the nature of the objects beyond describing what they look like. That is, they name and identify objects not according to their generation or cause (i.e., how they come to be), but according to how closely they fit a prototype. But the descriptive criteria may be arbitrary—chosen as they are by interested parties—so that the objects encompassed by them may be close or distant in nature (i.e., the distinctions being artificial).

A field guide system working with appearances (and without any other reference to nature) is not constrained in the groups or classes it identifies. On the one hand, it can overexpand a group by encompassing many diverse individuals who share some superficial attribute. And on the other, it can multiply groups by making too much of trivial distinctions between individuals.

As a "field guide" for psychiatrists, *DSM* has brought both the strengths and vulnerabilities of this approach to them. It at least temporarily settled many arguments over diagnostic terminology and usage. And it certainly provided the reliable identifications needed to launch and sustain research in a fashion unknown in psychiatry prior to its publication in 1980. For these achievements we are in its debt.

But the field guide method—so useful for research—is less useful in clinical practice, where it promotes the diagnostic misdirections and therapeutic rigidities that abound today, and does so by burdening practitioners with both of the standard problems of field guides. In *DSM* there are examples of overinclusion, in which patients of a motley kind are encompassed within a single diagnostic class: As well there are examples of artificial distinctions, such that many more classes of disorders than were ever imagined are now in *DSM-IV* or waiting in the vestibule. Let me expand on these points.

DSM forges an overinclusive category when, in choosing to emphasize some symptoms as dictating a diagnosis, it merges under a single heading very different patients (and nonpatients) and minimizes important distinctions in the nature and needs of individuals. Hence all the forms of sadness and dispiritedness to which humans are vulnerable tend to be wrapped within the *DSM* diagnosis "major depression," with the result that many patients are medicated (and overmedicated) rather than receiving more apt therapy and care for a sad state of mind tied to their social situations and life burdens.[2]

Overinclusive diagnoses pervade *DSM-IV*. Every restless child—especially if a boy—now comes under the shadow of attention deficit/hyperactivity disorder (ADHD) and faces Ritalin rather than recess to "cure" him. So many shy persons nervous about public speaking have been diagnosed with social phobia that its advocates hold that one in every eight Americans suffers from this "disorder." And any soldier who experiences mental disquiet will be fitted under the rubric of post-traumatic stress disorder (PTSD) no matter what other issues his or her life reveals.

The drawing of distinctions without differences explains why with each new edition of *DSM* (from *DSM-III* on) the number of "identified" psychiatric conditions has grown steadily, expanding the size of the manual from 119 pages before *DSM-III* to 886 pages in *DSM-IV*, with no limits in sight. Advocates have emerged with every iteration of the manual to propose new "disorders." A fresh candidate awaiting approval is caffeine withdrawal syndrome. And of course it was through eager advocates that MPD came to prominence in *DSM-III*.

Because they were drafting a field guide, the authors of *DSM-III* could not reject MPD when a number of psychiatrists claimed to be able to recognize the condition and were ready with "diagnostic criteria." (In fact, all psychiatrists now realize that in order to get a diagnosis into *DSM*, what is needed is a "political" ticket and a "claims" ticket—i.e., a sizable group of psychiatrists to "lobby" the APA for a diagnosis [the "political" ticket] all of whom agree on the set of defining symptoms [the "claims" ticket].)

The authors of *DSM* could not demand that the champions of MPD provide the nature, causes, or mechanisms of the disorder, given that such conceptual standards were not required of other disorders in the manual. The authors of *DSM-III* had proclaimed that their manual would function "a-theoretically." This meant (again, whether they understood it or not) that the authors were left without any checks on diagnostic classes that kept medical diagnoses from expanding without limit. *DSM* only demanded from those clamoring for the inclusion of a "disorder" that the symptoms presented as diagnostic criteria be sufficiently clear for psychiatrists to recognize them.

And so *DSM-III* embraced MPD. It listed the following three symptomatic "features" as diagnostic: (1) "existence within the individual of two or more distinct personalities," (2) "the personality that is dominant determines the individual's behavior," and (3) "each individual personality is complex and integrated with its own unique behavior patterns and social relationships." And, of course, being "a-theoretical," *DSM* made no judgment as to whether these features defined a real or artificial condition.

This explains why I regularly and confidently answer, "No," when facing the challenging question "If it's in *DSM-IV*, isn't it real?" I then try to teach how a history and a method worked their mischief.

MPD marched into *DSM-III* because of weaknesses built into the manual by the leaders of psychiatry who were preoccupied with a divisive historical moment in the discipline. Being listed in *DSM* tells one nothing of the objective existence of any disorder, including MPD. But that listing has given MPD (and its presumed mechanisms) a legitimacy that to this day is proving hard to curb.

And so when I'm asked another (perhaps more friendly) question, such as "Just how could this set of ideas about mental life, which will not bear much scrutiny, emerge within psychiatry and become so conspicuous?" I describe this outcome as a paradoxical and unintended consequence of a political effort at resolving controversy and promoting progress within psychiatry. The attempt to make clinical diagnosis reliable with a symptom-based field guide produced much good. It advanced research and improved consultations and communications over many psychiatric disorders. But, it provided an entree for many deceptive claims

The MPD story confirms the adage that the problems of today are usually due to the solutions of yesterday. In particular, it demonstrates how political pressure can force artificial conditions into *DSM*. This flaw in the system will persist until the field guide method of diagnosis in psychiatry is supplanted by a systematic one. Hurry the day, I say.

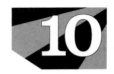

What Is Meant by
Hysteria?

As recounted earlier in this book, the journalist Flora Rhea Schreiber collaborated with Manhattan psychiatrist Cornelia Wilbur in writing *Sybil*, the story of the young woman who, over time while under Dr. Wilbur's care, developed sixteen "personalities." In each distinct "alter" guise she behaved in a different way—depicting aggressive males, defenseless children, and intellectual women at one time or another and often in succession.

In their book, the collaborating authors proposed that this "disintegration" of Sybil's mind into several personalities was the result of her "repressing" the memory of sexual abuse she suffered at the hands of her mother in childhood. Although the abuse was never confirmed, the book and the television movie made from it ignited the MPD craze.

After the book's publication, Schreiber heard from numerous women who credited her with opening their eyes to their own multiple personalities. Her book triggered other biographies of multiple personalities, only one of which—*The Minds of Billy Milligan* (1981)—remains in print. *Sybil* and these other books—which also linked MPD to childhood abuse—appeared at a time when much mistreatment of children was being confirmed with distressing and increasing frequency by pediatricians.

What went unmentioned in *Sybil*, though, was the serious difference of opinion between Dr. Wilbur and Dr. Herbert Spiegel about the patient herself. Dr. Spiegel is a psychiatrist who specializes in the study of hypnosis (and the father of Dr. David Spiegel, whom I mentioned earlier as an MPD advocate). He had been consulted by Dr. Wilbur about the use of hypnosis with Sybil. In an interview with historian Mikkel Borch-Jacobsen in May 1995,[1] Dr. Spiegel described how he came to know Sybil well, having examined her many times, and how he eventually told Wilbur and Schreiber, "She's not a multiple personality."

Spiegel defined Sybil as "a wonderful hysterical patient with role confusion, which is typical of high hysterics. It was hysteria."

Schreiber, though, rejected his interpretation "in a huff" and insisted that they must stick to the original diagnosis because "if we don't call [her] a multiple personality, we don't have a book! The publishers *want* it to be that, otherwise it won't sell!" (italics in original).

Dr. Spiegel, looking back at the publication of *Sybil*, commented on how it had started "a whole new cult, a whole new wave of hysteria restated in a new way. ... basically it's a hysterical response to hysteria." He believed that MPD therapists were "taking highly malleable, suggestible persons and molding them into acting out a thesis that they are putting upon them."

What, though, did Spiegel mean by the words he chose? Particularly what did he mean by *hysteria*? And what clinical and historical background was he drawing upon when he used the word to characterize both the patient he examined (the Ur-patient of the "recovered memories of sex abuse") and the events that followed the publication of *Sybil*?

In everyday use, *hysteria* and its adjective *hysterical* describe a state of being overly emotional, wildly dramatic, and behaving out of control. Although this usage is common enough (and Spiegel uses the adjective *hysterical* at least once in this way), psychiatrists using the term diagnostically mean something more specific than "overly emotional." And certainly I intended something quite specific when, testifying at the Danny Smith trial, I said his accusing daughter, Donna, suffered from hysteria.

By the diagnosis "hysteria," psychiatrists mean to identify a perverse human behavior in which the subjects act in ways that imitate physical or psychological disorders of a kind that draws medical and nursing attention to them. Those subject to the condition are always diagnostic challenges to physicians in that their behavioral mimicry of disease can be extraordinary. As Thomas Sydenham, the illustrious seventeenth-century physician, pointed out:

> This disease is ... remarkable for ... the numerous forms under which it appears, resembling most of the distempers wherewith mankind are afflicted. For in whatever part of the body it be seated, it immediately produces such symptoms as are peculiar thereto; so that unless the physician be a person of judgment and penetration he will be mistaken, and suppose such symptoms to arise from some essential disease of this or that particular part, and not from the hysteric passion.[2]

Physicians and surgeons often view hysterical patients with suspicion and disdain. When these doctors grasp the psychological rather than physical source of these puzzling complaints, they often presume some fraudulent intent on the patient's part. But psychiatrists hold that an essential feature of hysteria—that which lies behind the medically imitative behavioral displays—is a vivid form of *self*-deception rather than a swindle.

In conceiving the problem of hysteria this way, psychiatrists can assert that these patients, influenced as they are by social and psychological circumstances, sincerely believe they are in some way sick and act on that belief. The patients expect to be accepted as sick people by others, to be given those benefits of care and the privileges of social support the sick ordinarily receive; to be, in terms sociologists employ, admitted to "the sick role," where protection is offered and fewer demands are made. The key to understanding them (and ultimately helping them) is to appreciate how they are self-deceived rather than being in search of entitlements they don't deserve.

In identifying self-deception as a fundamental feature of hysteria, psychiatrists do not deny that some potential for self-deception is a universal, occasionally comforting, human characteristic—as represented, for example, in how any one of us can occasionally "forget" some onerous obligation, "ignore" a painful conflict, or "expect" more than we deserve. But with hysteria, psychiatrists identify the expression of this human capacity for self-deception in what may be its most radical form. And with the diagnosis, they begin to search for social, psychological, and even physical contributions promoting and sustaining the self-deceiving assumptions of the patient.

I followed this course when I defined Donna Smith as an example of someone who suffered from hysteria. I held that her beliefs that she had MPD were evoked by her therapist at a time in Donna's life when she was feeling discouraged and depressed. And then, when she was isolated from friends and family and secluded on a hospital ward specializing in MPD, her self-deception and her false memories were amplified and shaped into flagrant misconceptions about harboring many distinct personalities and being a victim of parental abuse and satanic rituals.

On that ward (and throughout her waking time), the psychiatrists and staff stressed that she was indeed "multiple," that her "abuse" was the most "real" aspect of her life, and that her inability to surrender completely to their ideas hindered the recovery she would gain by trying to remember what had "happened" to her.

When she was separated from these doctors and nurses, she promptly recovered herself, her grasp of reality, and the truth of her childhood—thus confirming the diagnostic opinion that her disorder was hysteria.

Clinicians recognize that hysteria is not something the patient has—like a rash or a fever—but is something the patient is doing. He or she is imitating a medical, surgical, or psychiatric disorder and thus will complain of subjective symptoms such as pains, faintness, or confusion, or will display physical signs such as seizures or paralysis. Hysterical patients complain dramatically and draw attention to their plight. One of the confusing aspects of hysteria is that patients may indeed already be genuinely sick, with such valid physical or mental ailments as epilepsy, toxicity, depression, and the like. So why act unwell on top of that?

It is the benefits, not the burdens, of being sick that such patients seek—especially greater concern, protection, and support. Even when already sick with some condition—and so perhaps weakened in their social judgment—they strive for more supportive attention.

Hysterical patients may come to believe that they are sick because of difficulties faced at work—difficulties that may be avoided by extending a hospital stay. They may be bewildered by a family conflict and assume the "sick role" in order to free themselves from obligations. Surprising as it may be, they seem willing—in exchange for small benefits—to accept life as an invalid.

Because hysteria is a behavior in which illness is imitated, patients with hysteria will always show symptoms that reflect the attitudes and beliefs about sickness held by the doctors who observe them. How else could they know about them?

The goal of appearing sick is not calculatedly chosen so much as it is gradually assumed when, through the interactions between patients and staff, advantages emerge, inferences are made, implications are noticed, and encouragement is received. The patients *learn* the behavior as they live and interact with others in a medical system.

Thus it is usual for a hysterical condition to progress from a beginning with minor complaints or weaknesses that then worsen until the features become incapacitating. The initial complaints are joined by other, more incapacitating complaints often inadvertently suggested and evoked by the interest and concern shown by an examining doctor.

This phenomenon—in the past described as the "incubation" of hysteria—usually indicates that the patients are gathering information about their "sickness." As mentioned, they are often responding to suggestions that the physicians, nurses, or other patients inadvertently supplied in the course of their assessment and care. But they may, in a state of worry, be consulting the Internet, which provides a vast wealth of information, such as how sicknesses present, what symptoms run together, and which attract prompt attention. Whatever the source (and it may be just seeing another person with symptoms), patients learn how their behavior affects others and then justify, mostly to themselves, the attention they are receiving by amplifying their symptoms and signs.

What precipitates hysterical behaviors? Occasionally, a dramatic, emotionally laden event such as a family crisis or a report of the death of an honored public figure such as Princess Diana or Pope John Paul II can provoke the sudden onset of hysterical paralysis, muteness, or fugue in a highly suggestible person. More often, hysterical conditions emerge in patients seeking care and support for some mixture of discouragement or demoralization tied to their temperament and life circumstances. Perhaps the patient senses and resents some lack of concern from others, or feels overwhelmed by responsibilities. He or she might feel unable to continue with military service or follow through on promises or expectations.

People vulnerable to hysteria are often emotionally if not chronologically immature and have regularly and habitually exaggerated or dramatized their feelings. They are also often highly hypnotizable, as Herbert Spiegel has stated.

Although the imitations of illness that hysterics display can be compelling, particularly if the patient is a nurse or doctor, progress in the basic skill of examining patients and the advances in technology over the past century have made many of these synthetic illnesses easier to identify as counterfeit: epileptic seizures occur without evidence of brain changes on the electroencephalogram (EEG); paralyses appear without any of the customary changes in the tendon reflexes (e.g., the knee jerk reflex); and faints and fugues are usually performed in ways that do not endanger the patient. Indeed, the dysfunctions of hysteria tend to be those that burden others—nurses, physicians, physiotherapists, and relatives—whereas symptoms that would burden the patient, such as urinary incontinence, tend not to occur.

If they win much public attention from their hysterical behavior, patients may hold on to it long after the circumstances that provoked it disappear. They can often be helped to let go of their symptoms if trusted doctors tell them ("countersuggest") that they are in the "recovery" phase of their "illness" and that the manifestations can be properly ignored, as they are but fading remnants of the resolving process.

Then, often to the surprise of all, many patients can abandon all the symptoms without doubting the validity of the original "sickness." This kind of face-saving helps resolve some clinical impasses that had been sustained by social factors.

Hysteria is not disappearing. It waxes and wanes in prevalence and how it manifests. Psychological guises, such as amnesias, fugues, and multiple personalities, tend to be more common today than neurological ones, such as seizures, paralyses, and sensory losses, that were in vogue a century ago. Psychological symptoms may be just more difficult to unmask.

Despite many efforts by psychiatrists to account for hysterical behavior by tying it to some specific underlying brain disorder—even using the functional brain imaging available today—none has succeeded. For this reason, the psychiatrist Thomas Szasz claimed in his famous antipsychiatry book, *The Myth of Mental Illness* (1961), that hysteria was not a "legitimate disease."

But psychiatrists do not see hysteria as a "disease," but as a behavioral disorder, one that they don't seek out but have imposed upon them, usually in their role as consultants to other physicians and to surgeons. It derives not from some change arising within a cell or neural pathway—from some identifiable pathophysiology, as in the case of diseases—but from some provocative events within the uniquely human world of self-consciousness. By this I mean that high level of mental functioning where one is aware of one's own individuality and where one's perceptions of reality can be powerfully shaken by social structures, language, and symbols.

Once one realizes that hysteria derives from what patients think and perceive about their lives and their world, it follows that the symptoms they display will most often reflect the ideas and assumptions held by people of influence in their culture. Today the influential leaders are doctors (psychiatrists even); in earlier times, they were clerics or teachers. A look back at historic mini-epidemics of hysteria demonstrates how collusions of attitude about health and sickness tied to persuasive authorities, unverifiable claims, and self-deceived subjects lay at the heart of what were often grim affairs.

Perhaps the best-known hysterical epidemic in America—the witch trials of Salem, Massachusetts—started when a group of girls between the ages of eleven and sixteen began to complain of pains, weakness, and rather melodramatic miseries that puzzled the local physician. He, unable to find a better explanation, stated that "the evil hand is on them" and referred the cases to the local magistrates and clergymen. He thought the girls might be victims of witchcraft.

The doctor had a clear enough concept: He, like everyone else in his society, believed that Satan, through the agency of his minions—witches and wizards—could distress and abuse people by, among other things, provoking illnesses and ailments. But the young girls whom the doctor identified as bewitched were also by his "diagnosis" licensed to accuse local citizens of being the witches who were torturing them in various ways—mostly by pinching and beating them, but also by appearing at night to wake them from sleep, frightening and threatening them.

The girls went along with the doctor's opinion and thought the dramatic behaviors they and their friends displayed—screaming from pain, falling to the floor shaking, twisting and contorting themselves—might be caused by some diabolical agent. Crucial and persuasive to the development of this story were the assumptions of the Salem community—including its magistrates—about the particular powers of witches.

Tradition held witches to be sly and deceptive—ever seeking to do harm. Also, people who were believed to be witches were thought capable of being in two different places at the same time (visiting and torturing girls in Salem at the very time they were seen meeting with friends in Boston) and able to provoke pain in a victim across the courtroom even while all eyes of the jury were on them in the dock.

These capacities, almost everyone assumed, derived from the powers Satan provided the witch. And so, a person could be found guilty on evidence no one could disprove. This so-called spectral evidence drove the witch trials.

These and other assumptions were based on the claims of the many witch hunters of Europe of the sixteenth and seventeenth centuries. They had described the powers of witches and even offered "operational" means for recognizing them, such as by skin defects and freckles, thought to represent evidence of physical contact with the devil or his imps.

The civil responses in Salem and elsewhere combined religious and legal actions. The relief of the girls was sought through prayer in churches and through the indictment of the accused and execution of those who stubbornly would not "confess" to being witches.

When imprisonment or even execution of the supposed culprits did nothing to suppress the girls, when they began to accuse more citizens—including the wife of the governor of Massachusetts Bay Colony—those who had pointed out that no one could contradict spectral evidence began to be heard. It took much courage, though, to speak out against the beliefs and the evidence, because the outspoken often quickly joined the accused.

The accusing girls did not always receive support everywhere they went. On one noteworthy occasion, they had been summoned to testify in Gloucester, but on their way, while crossing a bridge in Ipswich, they passed by an old woman and promptly fell into their fits of screaming, falling, and twisting—accusing the woman of torturing them.

The townspeople of Ipswich were not impressed by these antics, as had been the villagers in Salem. They had not summoned the girls, thought little of their testimony and behavior, and simply ignored them as they lay on the bridge bellowing away.

The girls, unaccustomed to being neglected in this way, became confused but eventually recovered from their fits, remounted their horses, and quietly rode on to Gloucester. Their courtroom testimony there, however, "lacked its usual conviction and led to no arrests."[3]

Things quieted down, but talk continued about just what had happened. The Harvard professor Cotton Mather wrote a book about the Salem trials, *Wonders of the Invisible World* (1692), in which he dramatically indicted Satan and his supernatural powers. The book injured Mather's reputation in history. Although he did express some reservations about spectral evidence, he found no fault in its use in bringing indictment and death to many, including an old Harvard acquaintance, Reverend George Burroughs, who had been accused by the Salem girls of being a wizard. With Mather's encouragement, Burroughs was brought back from Maine, where he farmed and preached, and promptly tried and executed.

Governor Sir William Phips, whose wife had been accused, was not long of two minds about the matter, however. He requested and received a second opinion on witchcraft and its detection from a group of distinguished ministers in New York. Although they also believed in witches as people "throwing off the yoke of God," these consultants denied that simple rules existed for identifying them. The New Yorkers specifically condemned the use of spectral evidence, replying, when asked whether it could be trusted, "By no means!"

Governor Phips redefined what evidence could be brought against the accused and ruled out every "spectral" claim of being pinched and choked, paid ghostly visitations, or transported by witches. As a result, all subsequent accusations collapsed.

Those who had previously "confessed" could be legally punished, but after the governor learned that the evidence brought against them was no different from that used against those who had been cleared, he signed reprieves for all and released them from prison. No one listened to the girls again.

Eventually several of the girls retracted their accusations. In 1706, one of the leading girls, Ann Putnam Jr., stood tearfully in the Salem Village church and in front of a congregation that included relatives of victims of her false charges listened as her minister read out her confession to them. In it she said how she wished "to be humbled before God … in that I was a cause with others of so sad a calamity. It was a great delusion of Satan that deceived me in that sad time. … I did it not out of any anger, malice, or ill-will."

One of the judges, Samuel Sewall, realized how he had contributed to these grim events and, also in church before his peers and neighbors, accused himself of "the blame and shame of it." And a minister, John Hale, who had testified against a woman subsequently executed, wrote to confess his errors: "We walked in clouds and could not see our way." He explained how "the lamentations of the afflicted and the power of former precedents" misled him.

The craze was over in Salem. It lasted little more than a year, but during its reign twenty people had been executed and more than a hundred imprisoned. But it was ended locally, relatively quickly in comparison with other crazes, and did not spread from Massachusetts.

Some credit can be given those like Judge Sewall and Reverend Hale, who acknowledged their errors, and some blame can be attached to Cotton

Mather, who, despite his doubts, never used his intellectual gifts and prominence to stop the craze. Although a few other witch trials had preceded it, the Salem incident was the last in colonial America and among the last of the witch persecutions anywhere in the Western world. They had gone on in Europe for over two hundred years—the last legal execution for witchcraft occurred in Glarus, Switzerland, in 1782. With the emergence of commitment to the natural sciences during the eighteenth century, the idea of devils and supernatural powers holding humans in their control was debunked.

But the replacement of a spiritual worldview with scientific positivism and empiricism did not end the human capacity for entertaining and promoting beliefs capable of generating hysterical behaviors. Several other historical examples demonstrate that any view of the world is capable, under certain circumstances and with the right advocates, of breeding the self-deceptions and behavioral misdirections of hysteria.

A fine example followed the arrival in sophisticated prerevolutionary Paris of Franz Anton Mesmer, who arrived from Austria in 1778 armed with a conception of nature that he claimed illuminated the physical basis of terrestrial existence and life itself. He proposed that a superfine invisible fluid surrounded and penetrated animate and inanimate objects. This hypothetical energy-bearing fluid, he taught, permeated heat, light, electricity, gravity, and magnetism—all the physical phenomena under study by the scientists of the times.

Mesmer was a physician and developed his ideas further as patients were drawn to him and his method of treatment. He taught that sickness was caused by some "block" to the flow of this energetic fluid through the human body (which he likened to a magnet). He claimed that he could unblock this flow by massaging the body with magnets and other metallic devices at the body's "magnetic poles."

These treatments occasionally "provoked" a remarkable attack or "crisis" in which the patient fainted or convulsed as the "energy" flow was restored. And, so Mesmer observed, on passing through this crisis the person was often refreshed and restored once again to "harmony" with nature.

For close to a decade, the flamboyant Mesmer enjoyed great success in Paris and gathered considerable wealth from supporters of his concepts as well as from patients he treated. Much of his success can be tied to how he treated distressed and discouraged people, brought hope that their conditions were susceptible to his care, and persuaded them ultimately to testify to his good effects on them.

Mesmer encouraged his patients to perform to his commands. His reputation for remarkable powers—of getting the blind to see, the deaf to hear, and the voiceless to sing—went before him as he proceeded in dramatic fashion to treat those seeking his care.

His treatment sessions were group affairs in which patients with such complaints as loss of energy, vigor, libido, and the like would sit together around a large vat of "magnetized," slightly acidified water holding to or leaning against iron rods that emerged from the vat and were meant to bring the magnetic energy to them and their afflicted bodies. As Henri Ellenberger points out, this contraption was a crude imitation of the recently invented (1746) Leyden jar for storing static electricity.[4]

With music playing in the room, Mesmer or one of his associates would approach the patients one by one, hold their hands, and prod their abdomens. Sitting quietly, listening to the music, and touched by the bars and occasionally by Mesmer, the patients reported a variety of inner feelings—of energy, of electricity, of rushing fluids—and many of them, at first singly but then often in a wave spreading across the group, would fall into a spell of convulsions (the "crises") and be carried convulsing from the room by Mesmer's burly attendants to recover. They claimed to feel better after this experience, which many likened to the old religious practice of exorcism.

Mesmer's patients were captivated not only by his appearance and his kindly, encouraging interactions with them, but also by the physical instruments he used and the scientific-sounding explanations of his treatments. His "success" he related to the invisible forces that, like the gravity of Isaac Newton and electricity investigated by Benjamin Franklin, worked their physical power most mysteriously.

That animal magnetism was but another kind of "spectral" proposition not so obvious to Mesmer's public and professional contemporaries. But in 1784, a Royal Commission led by Antoine-Laurent de Lavoisier (the great French chemist, discoverer of oxygen) and Benjamin Franklin (at the time the American ambassador to France and a well-known figure in Paris) concluded that Mesmer's clinical powers rested on his skills with suggestion and on the vivid imagination and readiness for self-deception of his clientele. The report noted that Mesmer's concept of animal magnetism had no material or scientific foundations, being rather a pseudoscientific conception that drew on analogies rather than true links with nature or science.

Again many people had taken up behaviors derived from a belief system that had come to prevail in their culture. The attention they received and the encouragement that came with it won their trust in the treatment and led them to imitate each other in its course. Their self-deception rested upon a concept that was unverified—animal magnetism—but derived a ring of validity from the intellectual framework of the times.

Even the debunking Royal Commission report did not end the matter. Mesmer did leave Paris soon after it came out, but his concepts of "magnetism" and "mesmeric healing" remained on the fringes of medicine until late into the nineteenth century. Even today, one meets people who believe that a few magnets in your shoes can do you good.

Mesmer was not a charlatan or fraud but a persuasive believer in his "system." His type is well known in medicine. Even in the contemporary world, figures emerge who claim to have some special knowledge about how to live life better and more healthily. They gain devotees and disciples through television, celebrity advocates, and advertising.

They often develop their ideas from extensions of current science and exotic philosophy and usually emphasize matters such as nutrition, "stress reduction," or cultural change. The leaders of these movements are, like Mesmer, of honorable intent and often comfort or heal by being responsive to the worries and misery of the patients they meet (who may well have been treated indifferently and unsympathetically by their physicians). But like him, they are usually stronger in charm and charisma than in accomplishment.

And occasionally, again like Mesmer, they can start up fads that have a hysterical aspect. Many of them draw on non-Western sources for their inspiration. The contemporary enthusiasm for the traditional Chinese medicine resuscitated by Mao and characterized by acupuncture and the "flow of chi" through the body in meridians and channels most startlingly resembles Mesmer's claims that sickness results from an obstacle to the flow of animal magnetism's superfine fluid through the body.

A third historical example of a mini-epidemic of hysteria is one I mentioned earlier. It, however, emerged not from the charisma of a "healer," but from the thinking of one of the most illustrious and capable neurologists (and a pioneering neuroscientist) of the mid-nineteenth century.

Jean-Martin Charcot brought "clinical-pathologic correlation" to the study of neurologic diseases. By that I mean he linked the symptoms and signs of illness that patients displayed in life to the specific changes in brain tissues found postmortem that must have caused those symptoms. In this way he differentiated and made sense of complicated and baffling neurological symptoms and disorders. He possessed the patience and skills of a perceptive clinician, and an enthusiasm for the study of the gross and microscopic changes he found in the brains of those patients he had carefully examined in life.

He conducted fundamental investigations into normal and pathologic anatomy and described for the first time many neurologic disorders. He was the first to recognize amyotrophic lateral sclerosis. This condition, referred to as Lou Gehrig's disease in the United States because it afflicted the famous New York Yankee baseball player, is known as Charcot's disease to this day in most of Europe. Similar eponymous clinical phenomena include Charcot's triad in multiple sclerosis, Charcot's joint in tabes dorsalis, and Charcot-Marie hereditary amyotrophic degeneration.

He made contributions to neurology at every level of complexity: conceptions of the organization of the cerebrum, the pathways in the spinal cord, and the functional responsibilities of peripheral nerves. He was "The Master" for most of the aspiring neuropsychiatric clinicians of Europe in his time and is recognized now as the founder of the great French tradition in neurology and neuropsychiatry.

Neurologist Israel S. Wechsler went even further, writing, "Of Charcot it may be said with truth that he entered neurology in its infancy and left it at its coming of age, largely nourished by his own contributions." The names of his students—Joseph Babinski, Georges Gilles de la Tourette, Pierre

Marie, Pierre Janet, Albert Gombault, Théodule Ribot, and others—grace the history of the discipline.

The epidemic of hysteria emerged when patients under his supervision at the Salpêtrière Hospital began to display convulsive contortions of their bodies during his rounds. A prior administrative decision played an inspiring part in these events; a reorganization of the clinic had put patients with episodic emotional disturbances on the same ward with epileptics. As the former witnessed the epileptic attacks and observed Charcot and his pupils so carefully studying the seizures and their effects, they began to display similar and even more remarkable symptoms and signs.

Charcot believed that he was observing—as he had on other occasions—an overlooked condition and began to devote much time examining the patients with this strange disorder. He thought he found distinct diagnostic signs, such as the "hand positions" the patients struck during their attacks, and concluded that, like the epilepsy patients with whom they were sharing a ward, they must have some physiologic defect provoking their condition. He began to refer to the condition as hystero-epilepsy, worked to distinguish it from other forms of epilepsy, and attended to the nuances of each case.

Over time, the numbers of patients with these symptoms gradually grew, new constellations of spasms and convulsions developed among them, and more and more of the staff became attentive to them. Charcot presented cases to observers in lecture halls open to the public and began to use the patients as subjects for the study of hypnosis. Their displays grew wilder as Charcot's interest in them increased.

But one of Charcot's most distinguished pupils, Joseph Babinski, began to suspect that the symptoms had been suggested to the patients by the clinical examinations that were repeatedly performed on them. Babinski thought that the patients had come to believe in their illnesses primarily because Charcot believed in them.

Charcot, on the other hand, presumed some brain source for the disorder. He was not dismayed by the lack of evidence for brain disease, because, he noted, many patients with other forms of epilepsy also have no evidence of brain pathology. Charcot (primarily on his authority as a great professor) could propose some mysterious pathology without fear of contradiction.

Eventually, as Babinski found support from Hippolyte Bernheim, a distinguished professor of internal medicine at the University of Nancy who also believed that the Salpêtrière patients were following suggestions, Charcot began to pull back from his presumptions of a neuropathologic cause for hysteria. He started to recognize the contagion of mimicry that occurred in the group and that patients improved when isolated from others with similar symptoms and from doctors bearing suggestion.

But Charcot died before he could complete his reassessment. His successor, Fulgence Raymond, believing that the hysterical symptoms were quite simply counterfeit, withdrew all attention to them. The patients ceased demonstrating the behaviors and the wards emptied out.

For all that this mini-epidemic of hysteria is interesting in itself, its subsequent effects on thought and practice are even more important. Two different clinical investigative paths in neurology and psychiatry emerged from Charcot's clinic.

The most direct path—essentially opened by Babinski—was to see the paralyses, seizures, and other antics of these patients as a manifestation of their self-deceptions and vulnerability to persuasion. Babinski emphasized how the symptoms were human creations—"artifacts" produced by contagion among the patients and by suggestion from Charcot's examination methods.

Following this line of reasoning, Babinski tried to help the patients recover by turning his attention away from the hysterical symptoms, offering realistic countersuggestions, and assisting the subjects in dealing with any present and provoking distress. His was a treatment based on what he saw going wrong. If persuasion could produce the disorders, then counterpersuasions could cure them, he thought. It seems a sensible idea.

The other path from Charcot's clinic was that followed by Sigmund Freud, who studied under Charcot from October 1885 through February 1886 (a total of four and a half months). They became friends, and eventually Freud translated two of Charcot's influential texts into German (*New Lectures on the Diseases of the Nervous System, Especially Hysteria* and *Clinical Lectures*).

Freud was captivated by Charcot and particularly with Charcot's interest in the use of hypnosis with hysteria to draw out memories of past events. In his obituary of Charcot, Freud claimed for him "the glory of being the first to elucidate hysteria."

But Freud rejected any idea of a mysterious neuropathology in these patients. He turned to proposing hidden psychological mechanisms—equally impossible to prove or disprove—as the best explanations for the hysterical displays of the patients and the critical mechanisms to address for their recovery.

Back in Vienna with Josef Breuer, he studied the case of Anna O., a young woman of considerable intellectual ability but with complicated and changing hysterical symptoms. Through their collaboration over this case, Freud and Breuer came to the idea that some kind of traumatic memories haunted all patients with hysteria and that the patients needed to have these memories "swept away" by talking them through, ideally under hypnosis. "Hysterics suffer mainly from reminiscences" was the aphorism Breuer and Freud advanced.

It is remarkable (even breathtaking) to realize that despite all the changes in theory and practice that Freudian psychoanalysis underwent over the following decades, this basic idea—one heals by remembering—has never been questioned. It remains today as the fundamental concept behind the MPD and recovered memory craze.

What do these three classical examples of hysteria have in common? And how do they resemble the recent outbreak of MPD hysteria? These similarities are easily enumerated.

First, the subjects in all these outbreaks of hysteria were "true believers"—they believed they were bewitched, mesmerized, or seizure-prone. In just the same way, patients with MPD believe they are "multiples."

Second, the patients' beliefs derived from conceptions of reality held by others and particularly by influential others—the doctors and divines of Salem, Mesmer and his distinguished supporters in Paris, Charcot ("The Master") at the Salpêtrière. In the same way, the patients with MPD derive their beliefs from the conceptions of mental life held by therapists to whom they entrust themselves.

Third, the belief-generated behaviors spread among subjects and grew in intensity with each individual: the girls in Salem grew more violent in their attacks and wider ranging in their accusations; the patients of Mesmer fell into waves of "crises;" the Salpêtrière women began to enhance their behaviors in steadily more dramatic ways. All of them were learning the behaviors that would draw and sustain attention from others.

And so with the MPD and recovered memory hysteria, once a single alter is found, more and more can be expected to appear, so that eventually hundreds may well emerge. The false memories begin as vague suspicions and then, being cultivated, grow to wild claims of abuse, including being a victim of satanic rituals and international, transgenerational conspiracy cults.

Fourth, the more attention paid to a behavior, the more the behavior was seen; the less attention paid, the less it was seen: the Salem girls found the magistrates' attention rewarding but the townspeople's neglect on the Ipswich bridge disconcerting and disempowering; Mesmer's patients had crises under his eyes and with his touch, but these crises disappeared with his departure from Paris. Charcot could get more behavioral displays with more exhibitions, while Raymond, his successor, ended the epidemic by refusing all attention. With MPD, more attention produces more alters, whereas no attention leads to the disappearance of the behavior. Many stories similar to that of Donna Smith's recovery from MPD after leaving her treatment team at Sheppard Pratt continue to be told—the most common being of patients who recover within a week or two after being transferred (usually because their health insurance ran out) from expensive MPD clinics to state hospitals, where their MPD symptoms were essentially ignored.

What can we finally say about these recurrent epidemics of imitative physical and mental disorder—in particular what agency transmitted the contagion from patient to patient? The transmission is quite simply through words—persuasive words and often ambiguous words. Patients with hysteria, whatever else they bring in the form of personal vulnerabilities and distressful states of mind, are expressing in their actions what they first heard about through influential words.

Words channel meaning, direct patients into behavioral displays, and to a most remarkable degree promote in the champions of these disorders the confidence that sustains their powers of persuasion. Because hysteria is a disorder that depends on words—words that describe, explain, bewitch, persuade, blind, convince—it is to the words about hysteria that we now must turn in this effort to make sense of these misdirections of concept and practice.

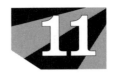

Words, Words, Mere Words

Almost all psychiatrists know (and some can even recite) the following whimsical passage from Lewis Carroll's *Through the Looking Glass*, which involves making words do what you want them to do:

> "I don't know what you mean by 'glory,'" Alice said.
>
> Humpty Dumpty smiled contemptuously. "Of course you don't—till I tell you. I meant 'there's a nice knock-down argument for you!'"
>
> "But 'glory' doesn't mean 'a nice knock-down argument,'" Alice objected.
>
> "When *I* use a word," Humpty Dumpty said, in a rather scornful tone, "it means just what I choose it to mean—neither more nor less."

> "The question is," said Alice, "whether you *can* make words mean so many different things."

> "The question is," said Humpty Dumpty, "which is to be master—that's all."

Psychiatrists occasionally refer to this passage when describing their work with stubborn patients or difficult bureaucrats. Never, though, was it more apt than in the MPD dispute, where words like *hysteria, repression, dissociation, personality, identity,* and the like were used with special and often changing meanings.[1] Here, in a time of science triumphant, what psychiatric authorities said, believed, and did powerfully affected how patients were thought of and treated.

The word *hysteria* itself has long been out of favor. Its etymological connection with the uterus (*hysteron* is the Greek word for uterus) derives from the ancient, condescending, and rightly discredited idea that uterine disorders—read female sexual problems—explain it. Psychiatrists naturally would prefer some term that speaks to its true nature—a mimicry of disability resting on self-deception and responsive to persuasion.

Most proposals to replace *hysteria* with terms that might grasp these essentials and indicate what lies behind its multifarious clinical presentations have not won support. Joseph Babinski proposed the term *pithiatism,* which means "cure by persuasion" (emphasizing how hysterical patients respond), and the contemporary British psychiatrist Harold Merskey coined the term *doxogenic,* which means "produced by opinion" (emphasizing how the symptoms depend on the patient's thinking and beliefs).

The authors of *DSM-III* ignored these interesting (and I think valuable) ways of finding a better diagnostic term for hysteria—again because they were, in principle, committed to using clinical appearances rather than any theoretical or generative concepts in their manual. But in striving to discriminate distinct categories of "appearances" in the disorder (which itself is the Monarch of Appearance and where appearance follows fashions) and to find terms for these different "appearances," *DSM* actually brought more confusion into the discipline and helped accelerate the MPD misadventure in clinical thought and practice.

DSM-III/IV divides the class of hysterical disorders into two groups based on the symptoms displayed by patients. It places all individuals who present physicians with complaints such as muteness, blindness, deafness, paralysis, or seizures (i.e., hysteria expressed physically) into the group labeled "conversion disorder," and all individuals who present physicians with complaints such as amnesia, perplexing unrecollected fugue-like wandering from home, or multiple personality (i.e., hysteria expressed psychologically) into the group labeled "dissociative disorder."

A mischief of meaning promptly sprang up around the words *conversion* and *dissociation*. And that mischief came through their derivations from past psychiatric theories.

The term *conversion* derives from the Freudian explanation of hysteria. Freud held that hysterical features of a physical kind (paralyses, seizures, blindness, etc.) result from the transformation, or "conversion," of the patient's repressed psychological conflicts into physical symptoms and manifestations.

His student Otto Fenichel described Freud's idea thus:

> Conversion symptoms are not simply somatic expressions of affects [i.e., emotions] but very specific representations of [unconscious] thoughts which can be retranslated from their "somatic language." ... [Hysterical] spells are pantomimic expressions of sometimes rather complicated fantasy stories. ... They represent distorted expressions of the Oedipus complex and of derivatives of the Oedipus complex. Sometimes the spells clearly betray that they stand for a sexual gratification.[2]

Although with the decline of Freudianism one might expect the concept of conversion to disappear, the word persists as a vestigial element in psychiatric parlance, replacing *hysteria* when identifying patients with quasiphysical symptoms. No one any longer believes that the hysterical patient's physical display represents symbolically his or her unconscious conflicts over sexual gratification. But for psychiatrists who hate the word *hysteria*, *conversion* can serve by agreement to identify physical phenomena—such as pseudoseizures or pseudoparalyses—generated by any sort of psychological unrest and sustained by self-deception.

If, however, *conversion* means the transforming of psychological problems into physical complaints, then *DSM-III* needed another term for the hysterical complaints that are themselves psychological, such as the fugues and MPD.

To serve these patients, the term *dissociation* (derived from another student of Charcot's hysterics, Pierre Janet) was resurrected. Janet, however, coined *dissociation* not solely for mental manifestations of hysteria, but to grapple with all hysterical phenomena. He claimed that *every* hysterical feature (physical and psychological) came from the patient's withdrawal of attention from some aspect of his or her "field of consciousness." By such withdrawal, parts of consciousness are cut ("dissociated") from willful or "self" control—either a part of consciousness responsible for the body (producing a weakness or paralysis in an arm or leg) or a part responsible for mental faculties (producing a loss of speech or memory). For Janet, there was no "conversion" in hysteria, there was only "dissociation."

To use Janet's own words, dissociation is "a retraction of the field of consciousness" so that functions such as movement, sensation, or memory are "dissociated from consciousness and therefore independent of its control (with resulting paralysis, anesthesia, or amnesia।"[3]

A moment's reflection reveals that this definition does not "explain" hysterical symptoms. Rather, it "describes" hysterical manifestations by means of a psychological metaphor. Dissociation is a "cutting," "retracting," "withdrawing" within "the field of consciousness," and as metaphor is a descriptive rather than explanatory term.

This fact in itself would be trivial if the word *dissociation* had not been put to use by clinicians with an axe to grind about memory and reality. In their hands—and with official *DSM-III* support for the dissociative disorder category—this descriptive metaphor carried unwarranted explanatory power into psychiatric practice.

Thus, *DSM-III*, in distinguishing by their manifestations the physical hysterias ("conversion symptoms") from the psychological hysterias ("dissociative symptoms") covertly implied that the two were different in nature. *DSM-IV* specifies that the complaints of patients with conversion disorders represent quasi- or pseudosymptoms and thus mimic disability. But *DSM-IV* also specifies that the complaints of patients with dissociative disorders represent actual rather than mimicked disabilities of mental faculties.

To quote directly from *DSM-IV*: "Conversion symptoms are related to voluntary motor or sensory functioning and are thus referred to as '*pseudo neurological*.'" On the other hand: "The essential feature of the Dissociative Amnesia is an *inability* to recall important personal information, usually of a traumatic or stressful nature … impairment in which memories of personal experience *cannot* be retrieved" (italics added).

Like Alice, we should ask "whether you can make words mean so many different things," given that the basic meaning of *hysteria* has long been the mimicry of illnesses and the artificiality of its manifestations. Clinical problems soon emerged in psychiatry with this kind of definitional mischief.

For instance, the assumption in *DSM-IV* that memory can be disabled led to Donna Smith's mistreatment. Her therapists could ignore her initial claim that she had no memory of being abused (a truthful claim, since she had not been abused) and presume that her powers of recollecting past "experiences" were impaired by dissociative amnesia. This justified their manipulative efforts to have her "try to remember" parental mistreatment and those satanic rituals they "knew" must be stored in her mind. With official, definitional support, these therapists never considered the possibility that they were suggesting rather than revealing past experiences to a sensitive and malleable subject—and thus inducing hysteria by producing quasi- or pseudomemories. They began with a case of depression and ended with a case of hysteria.

With these confusions of words, meanings, and assumptions about hysterical manifestations, many clinicians (including Herbert Spiegel, as noted previously) are, despite its awkward derivation, sticking with the original term, *hysteria*. Holding to *hysteria* seems no more unreasonable than holding to *schizophrenia*. Neither diagnostic term accurately describes the condition the patients suffer, but at least most of us know what we mean when we use it.

What remains to consider is an accounting of the extent of damage done (such as just how many people's lives were disrupted) by clinical practices resting on this particular example of hysteria, with its causal presumptions of hidden child abuse. The worst was the criminal prosecutions based on "repression" or "dissociation" of "memories" in children. Close to two hundred people like Kelly Michaels were prosecuted, many convicted and sent to prison, and some are still in jail today.

The number of adults in whom false memories were generated and who disrupted their families and lost their natural affections is more difficult to establish with confidence. But certainly there were many. In his fine book on the damage done to his own family by therapists, Mark Pendergrast estimates that during the few years of the explosive phase of this hysterical craze, some 1 million or so false memory cases were produced each year. He drew this conclusion from the number of practicing licensed therapists in the United States at the time (some 250,000), 25 percent of whom, based on the testimony of respondents in a 1994 survey carried out by Debra A. Poole and D. Stephen Lindsay, provided "memory-focused" therapies and claimed to recover memories in 34 percent of their approximately fifty female clients in a year (62,500 memory-focused therapists × 50 clients × 34 percent = 1,062,500 cases).[4]

This is obviously a rough estimate, but it does indicate the order of magnitude of the injuries produced by this craze. I presume that several million people were ultimately as severely affected as some of the patients I've encountered and described in this book. Certainly such numbers would explain why so many hospitals and clinics chose to build multiple personality services in the late 1980s and early 1990s. Institutions such as the Sheppard Pratt Hospital build only those programs for which they can anticipate a demand.

The FMSF stopped announcing the numbers of calls it received from families as those numbers approached 10,000, but it would say that some 25,000 families in one way or another have been in contact with the FMSF to find help in defending against recovered memory accusations. If one calculates that between five and ten people connected to each family (parents, children, siblings, grandchildren) would be affected by such a cruel accusation, again the magnitude of the injuries produced by the craze is vast.

I joined with several other members of the FMSF to attempt to document the characteristics of the people affected by false memories as well as other features of the recovered memory movement. Following is a summary of our study and its findings.

In 2001, we devised a questionnaire and sent it to 4,400 families who had contacted the foundation between its founding in 1992 and 2001. Of those questionnaires, 1,847 (of which 1,734 were informative) were returned (making the response rate 42 percent). The results helped us identify aspects of this craze that we had previously only presumed.

The accusers were essentially all Caucasian, 93 percent were female with a mean age of thirty-two years, and 77 percent were college graduates working in professional white-collar occupations. These demographics—highly educated, female dominant, upper-level occupational status—differ strikingly from those of the sexually abused but match the population features of people seeking psychotherapy. Indeed, 86 percent of these subjects were in formal psychotherapy when they made their accusations, and 48 percent had had previous mental disorders or illnesses.

The epidemic nature of the craze is evident when the dates of the first accusation are displayed. Accusations were rare in this group before 1985 but then grew exponentially, peaking in the years 1991–92, when 579 accusations (34 percent of total) were made. Thereafter, the number of accusations steadily declined, amounting to only 36 accusations (.02 percent of total) in 1999–2000.

Figure 11.1 shows the rise and fall of this craze. Given our findings, my colleagues and I saw only two possible explanations for why these adult women had accused their parents of abusing them in their early childhood: "Either an epidemic of child abuse and repressed memories occurred in the 1960s (in a population quite different from usual child molesters), or a craze in therapy occurred in the 1980s that afflicted many vulnerable and suggestible people only to be challenged, stigmatized and ultimately rejected when the damage was recognized. Surely the latter is more likely."[5]

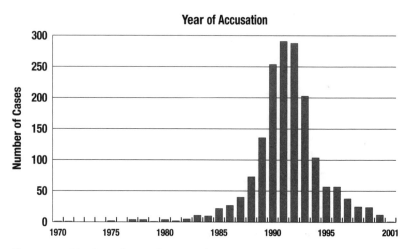

Figure 11.1. Number of cases by year of accusation. (*Source*: Paul R. McHugh, Harold I. Lief, Pamela P. Freyd, and Janet M. Fetkewicz, "From Refusal to Reconciliation: Family Relationships after an Accusation Based on Recovered Memories," *Journal of Nervous and Mental Disease* 192 [August 2004]: 525–31. Used with permission.)

But I took several other lessons away from this study and all that had come before it. In particular, I could say with even more confidence that the recovered memory craze of the 1980s and 1990s was not—as many wishing to avoid criticizing fundamentals of practice occasionally claim—simply an occasional lapse of therapists. It was far too extensive for that.

One also cannot view it as but a lapse in good practice distinct from the teaching of the psychiatrists who were its champions—a kind of slipup in the application of their ideas by the inexperienced. Had this been true, these ideas and their implications about the functioning of the mind would never have come to dominate leading centers of teaching and practice the way they did.

Indeed, the current mushrooming interest in post-traumatic stress disorder demonstrates how this misbegotten practice will evolve, as I will discuss in the next chapter. True believers have slowly shifted away from multiple personality disorder and renamed the associated problems PTSD or "betrayal trauma." The name changes, but what remains constant is an insistence that the mind processes trauma in a special way, and that memories of trauma can be encoded so differently from regular memories as to be inaccessible to consciousness unless prompted by such techniques as hypnosis or guided imagery.

Thanks to remarkable advances in memory science during the last decade, we can dismiss this purported psychological mechanism—call it "repression," "dissociation," or whatever. The work of Elizabeth Loftus, Richard Ofshe, and Richard McNally established both that testimony based on "recovered" memories cannot be trusted without corroboration and that the human mind has no specific tendency or ability to drive trauma from recall. As Richard McNally states unequivocally in his definitive book *Remembering Trauma*: "The notion that the mind protects itself by repressing or dissociating memories of trauma, rendering them inaccessible to awareness, is a piece of psychiatric folklore devoid of empirical support."

Surely McNally's stance makes biologic sense. If people tended to obliterate the memory of traumatic events, they would not learn from experience and would not avoid situations where trauma was likely to be repeated. A psychological inclination to forget traumas would jeopardize human survival.

Likewise, reasonable people should quickly grasp that a charge of sexual abuse alleged to have occurred years earlier based on recovered memories, and offered with no other corroboration but the view that "the mind works this way," renders everyone vulnerable to claims impossible to refute—like the spectral evidence of the Salem witch trials. Only Freud's long-standing influence in our culture and the subliminal suspicions it sustains about family life keep such obvious criticisms at bay.

Before we can be sure a similar persecutory psychiatry does not reemerge, this kind of thinking must be abandoned. But even the most thorough criticism and rejection of the ideas of the dynamic unconscious and repression seem unable to terminate these habits of thought amongst therapists.[6]

If misdirections of this sort are to be avoided, practicing psychiatrists and psychologists must turn away from "unconscious" mental mechanisms such as denial, repression, projection, dissociation, and the like that are as pliant as putty. Not only do these concepts of dynamic psychology encourage the composition of vivid "story explanations" of mental disorders, they discourage attention to other and simpler causes of mental distress.

Although therapists seem ever tempted to work like some latter-day Sherlock Holmes seeking a secret behind symptoms, these events teach that the search for the "hidden" and the "mysterious" is often a misdirection. It distracts therapists from straightforward empirical study of mental disorders and blinds them to how they may be suggesting the very symptoms they claim to be treating.

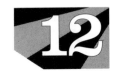

The Move to
Post-Traumatic
Stress Disorder

P sychiatrists promoting programs for multiple personality disorder
and searching for repressed memories of childhood sexual mistreatment found by the late 1990s that their work was proving a tricky
sell: the courts rebuked it, health insurance companies withdrew financial
backing for the prolonged hospitalizations prescribed, many malpractice
insurance policies specifically excluded their hypnotic induction practices,
and, with some protagonists speaking of satanic cults and ritualistic abuse,
many in the public saw much of it as fantasy. The promoters began to change
their tactics and reinterpret their ideas.

They never acknowledged that their methods of searching for memories
needed to be revised. And they certainly did not explain to their students
how the errors that provoked scandals of malpractice occurred. They never
repudiated their practices of generating arrays of alternative personalities in
their patients that attracted so much attention.

It was all a big misunderstanding, they said. All along, so they claim,
their intention was to show that the patients have personalities "fragmented"

rather than "multiplied" and are depressed or anxious because they cannot "integrate" the memory of their past traumatic experiences into their consciousness and life stories. Everything else, they want us now to know, was metaphor and not to be understood literally.

And so it happened that some time around the year 2000 the psychiatrists who had been most involved in the MPD work stopped emphasizing and collaborating with the vivid imagery of their patients' "multiplicity." They stopped talking to "alters" as if they were real, they gave up "charting alter relationships," and they stopped demonstrating how to use hand signals to evoke a silent "alter." Instead, they turned to using their suggestive methods to dredge up detailed and forgotten "traumatic memories" from their patients. They claimed they were attending more to what all their patients had in common—post-traumatic stress disorder (PTSD).

Just as they found a new diagnostic term for MPD patients, dissociative identity disorder (DID), they even changed the name of their group (now for the third time) from the International Society for the Study of Dissociation to the International Society for the Study of Trauma and Dissociation. These actions all served to call attention to their new goal of treating the various forms of PTSD and reconstituting minds shattered by "traumatic memories."

Did any of these rationalizations help patients? Not much. The treatments continued to be prolonged; the hunt for memories was carried out in the same way, with hypnosis, strong sedation, and suggestive probing; and many of the patients continued to be overly dependent on their therapists as they tried to remember the ostensible traumas provoking their symptoms.

But then PTSD is, and always has been, a most troubling diagnosis. Robert Spitzer, the main editor of *DSM-III*, recently observed, "Since [PTSD's] introduction into *DSM-III* in 1980, no other *DSM* diagnosis, *with the exception of Dissociative Identity Disorder* (a related disorder), has generated so much controversy in the field as to the boundaries of the disorder, diagnostic criteria, central assumptions, clinical utility, and prevalence in various populations" (italics added).

So why did the programs interested in searching for lost memories turn as one in its direction? They were drawn to it because patients given the diagnosis of PTSD had, by definition, suffered some traumatic experience and so therapists would be justified in searching for it.

And with predictably sad consequences, these "traumatologists," using this diagnostic concept and ever searching for hidden memories, would once again pass over crucial distinctions in their patients, exaggerate the role of trauma in their lives, and greatly complicate their care. They made mysterious what is actually straightforward.

PTSD is not a separate "entity" or "malady," but a natural emotional response provoked by frightening events and varying in its intensity from patient to patient depending on several factors. It is one of several kinds of human emotional distress that fall within the class of "emotions of adjustment"—a class that includes grief, homesickness, and certain forms of demoralization tied to rivalry or jealousy.

What is striking about all these emotions of adjustment is how similar they are to one another. Although we distinguish them by their causes and identify how loss produces grief, displacement produces homesickness, and threat produces PTSD, as states of mind they resemble each other so closely that without knowing how they came to be, they are difficult to tell apart.

Inevitably they will be mixed up when patients are diagnosed by symptoms alone—as of course *DSM-III/IV* demands. For example, all of them tend to generate vivid mental imagery and distressful dreams amounting to nightmares. All produce distracting thoughts, difficulty concentrating, diminished personal interests, and general misery. All can have physical components—trembling, loss of appetite and body weight, diarrhea, even hair loss. These symptoms often lead one to think some physical disease is at work.

Certainly patients who have experienced both the response to threat and the grief from loss are surprised by their similarity. C. S. Lewis, in describing his state of mind after the death of his wife, wrote: "No one ever told me that grief felt so like fear. I am not afraid, but the sensation is like being afraid. The same fluttering in the stomach, the same restlessness, the yawning. I keep on swallowing."

These emotions of adjustment usually remit with time, even though some features can continue long after the provocative events or distressful experiences. A piercing reminiscence can evoke a welling up of tears decades after the death of a beloved parent. And almost every serious college student, years after graduation, reports having the occasional dream in which he or she faces a crucial academic test or examination unprepared.

Each of these emotive states is customarily viewed as normal in that each is evoked in everyone under the right circumstances, tends to run a similar course, and seems "species specific" in that all who are subject to one of them describe much the same state of mind. Each is, though, graded in degree, can be disabling when extreme, and can be helped with treatment.

Psychiatrists do speak of "atypical" or "morbid" grief, homesickness, and jealousy and intend by those adjectives to identify how an emotion of adjustment can overrun its customary limits by extending far longer than is usual, by displaying unusual symptoms, and by blighting all social and occupational life. Then they must decide whether the atypical case represents the appearance of an additional disorder such as major depression, or the exaggerated way that the afflicted individual by temperament manages all emotional expressions. Clinicians make these distinctions every day.

The graded intensity of the emotions of adjustment depends upon matters tied to the provocative event, such as the severity of the readjustment demands, the availability of support and help, and the long-term implications of what happened. Losing a cherished child produces a greater grief than the loss of an elderly and long infirm parent. Moving alone to a foreign country where language, customs, cultural expectations, and professional demands are unknown produces a greater sense of dislocation and more persistent misery than moving with a family to another city in one's own country.

Supportive leadership in facing a disaster, personal characteristics of maturity and vision, financial means, and social stability are features that reduce the intensity of emotions of adjustment in that they strengthen the subject's ability to bring about a good result. The sense of loss of control is common to all these patients, even though it tends to be emphasized by champions of PTSD.

Although all these emotions of adjustment ordinarily settle with time and the patients adjust in some way to new circumstances, in their more prolonged and exaggerated forms they can provoke behaviors (such as alcohol consumption, aggression, or suicide), other mental illnesses (such as major depression), and even physical conditions (such as asthma).

But they are specifically *not* disorders of memory. Memories may shape some aspects of the impact of the provocative event—identifying, in relation to the new demands, all that was lost, settings to be missed, and past securities to be foregone. To steal from Marshal McLuhan, memory is the medium, not the message. And, as it turns out, memory is far from a reliable medium, not because experiencing losses or traumas drives the causes from memory (as the concept of "traumatic memory" can claim) but because the intensity of present emotions (and sometimes the suggestions of caregivers) can alter what is "remembered" and "believed." Experienced psychiatrists have often commented on how different—and usually worse—one's past life can seem when called to mind during a distressful emotional reaction.

And so to repeat for emphasis, PTSD is not a disorder of memory, nor is it caused by some failure of memory. Rather, with its symptoms of fear and dread, it is one of the normal emotions of adjustment. The key to helping patients experiencing any of these emotions of adjustment (and especially PTSD) is threefold. First, the symptoms should be seen for what they are—normal human reactions varying in severity depending on the individual and the contexts. Second, the patients should be treated by supportive management and coherent symptom relief, all with the aim of facilitating the recovery that will eventually emerge. Third, these conditions should be differentiated from and not confused with other emotional or behavioral conditions that can imitate them or emerge from them, including the major mental illnesses, personality disorders, or long-standing behavioral problems that demand treatment programs of their own.

But how has knowledge of the emotional responses to traumatic circumstances emerged, and how does that information confirm the idea that we are dealing with an emotion of adjustment in a patient? Psychiatrists have learned about the psychological responses to trauma from a century of caring for people shocked, injured, and terrified by perilous and horrific circumstances. Clinical opinions based on these experiences evolved mostly ad hoc, on the job, or retrospectively. And although important work was done and progress was made, as I'll describe, the process has proven difficult and many of the claims have been influenced by political, social, and even military considerations.

Psychiatric epidemiologists have carried out several recent "prospective" studies, the results of which have enhanced our grasp of the nature of the emotional responses to threat and trauma. In prospective studies, people who were exposed to known and documented traumatic experiences were followed up right after the initial trauma and examined over time to observe the emotional effects of the experiences and reveal what helps or hinders recovery.

Basically, all these studies indicate that traumatic experiences are common in human lives and that the emotional reactions reflect less the severity and nature of the trauma and more the resilience of the subjects and the management of the situations—as might be expected for emotions of adjustment.

A superb study was done by David Alexander, a psychiatrist in Aberdeen, Scotland. He studied the traumatic experiences and emotional reactions of a team of police officers involved in the salvaging of bodies from the North Sea after the 1988 disastrous explosion that destroyed the oil rig Piper Alpha.[1]

The dormitory module of the rig was recovered from the seafloor some months after the explosion. From this module and its surrounds, some seventy-three bodies were recovered—all in very deteriorated condition. The police searched for bodies in the refuse and helped bring them to the mortuary, where they were washed, photographed, and pathologically studied. This most grim and distressful experience had varying psychological effects on the men, which were carefully studied and followed over time by Dr. Alexander and his team.

By a remarkable piece of epidemiological luck, shortly prior to the disaster Alexander had assessed many of the same policemen and carried out several standardized measurements of their psychological status and mental characteristics. Thus he could compare their mental states and test responses before and after the disaster.

Many concepts about the meanings of disaster and emotional distress were brought to light by Alexander. Although all of the policemen were disturbed by these shocking experiences, they were emotionally comforted and did best when their leaders reminded them of the value of their work. These leaders repeatedly pointed out to them just how their efforts brought settled finality and some comfort to the families by rescuing the remains of their loved ones from anonymity and the cold sea. In this way, Alexander demonstrated how "role induction" for many grim enterprises has great value in preparing and supporting people as they face threats and traumas by affecting how they respond in the moment and how they think about their experience afterward. A failure to provide adequate role induction probably explains why many of the workers dealing with body recovery at Ground Zero in Manhattan after 9/11 experienced emotional distress that in some reached disabling levels.

The other results of Alexander's work are equally interesting. They revealed that most of the policemen in his study had distressful emotions of shock and fear but that everyone—doctors and subjects alike—saw these emotional states as normal and ones they could bear and recover from. Those policemen who had been identified in psychological testing as having high "neuroticism" scores (and so were constitutionally liable to react to events with more intense emotions) did suffer greater emotional reactions to their experiences than the others, but even they were not incapacitated by their feelings. None of the policemen was thought to be abnormal or labeled a PTSD patient.

An almost identical study to that of the Piper Alpha disaster—without the extra refinement of Alexander's pre- and postdisaster comparisons—was that of A. C. McFarlane in a group of firefighters involved in a terrifying and extensive Australian brushfire brought on by a prolonged drought in 1983.[2] The firemen were followed over the next thirty months with standardized psychological assessments.

As at Piper Alpha, the men all worked together and could corroborate all the experiences so that the observational facts about the nature of the threatening events were never in dispute. It is worth noting, however, that the firemen's individual self-reports of the events and the threats they faced often differed from more objective assessments of their encounters available through multiple informants—again confirming the crucial importance of verification when trauma histories are gathered.

The follow-up studies revealed that the dangerousness or hazard in the traumatic experience was not a crucial factor in any psychological reactions that ensued. Some firefighters became distressed with little threatening exposure, and some who went through the most terrifying of experiences suffered no lasting effects.

A third, more recent and most telling piece of prospective research was the study published in 2007 of a representative sample of 1,420 children from western North Carolina followed annually from ages nine to sixteen to see how often any of them experienced a traumatic event and what, if any, mental disorders followed. Over two-thirds of the children reported exposure to one or more traumatic events. Although what constituted trauma was broadly interpreted in this study, few subsequent symptoms were observed in most of the individuals and less than 0.5 percent of these children developed the symptoms of PTSD.

Those children with multiple traumas who lived under conditions of severe family adversity or who suffered from other psychiatric disorders were much more likely to suffer from depression and anxiety. The author concluded that "in the general population of children, potentially traumatic events are fairly common and do not often result in PTS symptoms, except after multiple traumas or a [personal] history of anxiety."[3]

All these prospective studies support the view that the emotional reactions to trauma and threat are emotions of adjustment that can vary in intensity both because of how the threats were perceived and because of the personal vulnerabilities and resilience of the person involved. PTSD is not a distinct mental disorder, but an intense and prolonged expression of the normal human emotional reaction to trauma.

This is certainly not what is implied in *DSM-III/IV*, and not what has been taught by the "traumatologists" who run the "trauma services" that replaced the MPD services. From their viewpoint, PTSD is a discrete mental disorder derived from identifiable traumatic experiences. They believe that the "trauma memories" have been "dissociated" (that old Pierre Janet term) and are acting and will continue to act disruptively, generating symptoms of depression and anxiety along with other behavioral problems.

How did these ideas—so different from the emotional adjustment view of traumatic reactions—develop? They derive from the original battles that put PTSD into *DSM-III* in 1980 and promoted the opinion that the condition is a mental "disorder" or malady rather than an intense form of normal emotional responsiveness. These claims were promoted by politically motivated and well-organized psychiatrists who recognized the importance of gaining a *DSM* label for their opinions. The story is fascinating and involved, and the outcome is only now close to resolution after some thirty years of practice and reflection.

Since World War I, psychiatrists have recognized that terrifying experiences with or without physical injury produce in everyone a fairly stereotyped psychological state of distress. They demonstrated that the psychological reaction to traumatic experience follows a loosely staged course—a course marked by emotional states of mind that differ somewhat in nature and expression depending on whether the traumatic experience was a sudden one, such as an explosion, or an extended exposure to threatening stresses, as in a long military campaign.

A sudden shocking trauma produces in most people an initial period of emotional numbness and "depersonalization" (the psychiatric term for a disruption in the sense of the reality of oneself or one's conscious experiences) that might last hours or even several days. During this time, traumatized people can act purposefully and give the impression of self-control, but if asked they will report that they function with an inner "dreamlike" sense of what's happening about them. Others observing them may note a strange poverty of emotional expression up to and including facial blankness and delayed responsivity.

This stage gradually subsides in a matter of days, to be replaced by a longer-lasting period of anxiety and painful remembering that can include difficulty sleeping, nightmares, vivid waking images (which some call "flashbacks"), and a phobic avoidance of the places and activities associated with the trauma. Finally, just as with a course of grief, the most disturbing psychological symptoms gradually fade away, leaving the subject with some enduring sense of loss, the occasional bad dream, and perhaps some reluctance to revisit locations or arenas where the shock was experienced.

Gradual is the operative word here, because the course of recovery can vary from days to months and depends on the severity of the trauma, its long-term implications, and the patient's own personality. But the key is that the reaction is normal and most people regain emotional equilibrium.

Most of the citizenry of New York City, all of whom had been exposed in one way or another to dreadful experiences on September 11, 2001, followed this course and recovered from the emotional turmoil of that day. Their steady mending surprised many contemporary "traumatologists" who had predicted a huge outbreak of PTSD among New Yorkers.

Differing from the emotional responses to an acute disastrous event are the characteristic emotional disruptions of those who live through extended periods of threat and traumatic encounters, such as soldiers in prolonged military campaigns. Under these circumstances, a more insidious mental condition—more a conditioned emotional state than an acute unconditioned response—can develop, especially if no respite from the assaults on body and mind is offered.

Everyone in such an unremitting stressful situation will eventually succumb to chronic anxiety and general ineffectiveness—again demonstrating these emotional reactions to be normal even as they appear in abnormal situations. This psychologically conditioned fearfulness will build slowly and may persist for weeks or months after an individual is removed from the stressful situation. However, it will ultimately dissipate, leaving some psychological remnants, such as the startle response many soldiers have to loud noises that resemble battlefield sounds (bangs, engine backfiring, sirens, etc.) or occasional vivid nightmares.

Psychiatrists consider the response to an acute traumatic event to be a straightforward unconditioned response, as specific to the event as is a startle response to a loud noise. In contrast, they consider the emotional condition that emerges from prolonged exposure to a threatening environment, as in trench warfare, to be more of a conditioned emotional state in which the subject has—as thousands of laboratory experiments in fear-conditioning documented—become physiologically reactive to the sounds and stimuli associated with the traumatic events in the environment.

As both reactions are expressions of emotions of adjustment, psychiatrists in the past expected their patients to recover as situations improved and adjustment was facilitated. And for the most part their expectations proved correct.

This standard concept took into account how aspects of situation, personality, and social role would shape both the acute and chronic forms of response, and it spoke to matters of individual vulnerability and resilience. It offered treatment and prognostic opinions that have stood the test of time and were neutral in judgment—neither denying the hero his laurel nor shaming the casualty with a white feather.

But these ideas of unconditioned and conditioned emotional responses to traumatic stress that made sense of combat soldiers' emotions of adjustment were pushed aside during and after the Vietnam War. At that point, certain psychiatrists began to advance the concept of PTSD as a kind of malady or distinct mental illness affecting memory and leading to emotional and behavioral disorders.

This concept was born through a partnership between some influential antiwar psychiatrists and a set of disturbed and distressed American veterans of the Vietnam War interested in emphasizing the cost of the war in human terms. They proposed PTSD as a special condition brought on by wartime experiences and causing a whole range of psychological ills that can last years—even decades—after the end of military service because of the "traumatic memories" that subsequently disrupt all of psychological life.

The history of this movement within psychiatry and its effect on diagnosis and treatment exemplifies perfectly how cultural attitudes and power politics can come to dominate the profession's assumptions about meaning, memory, and mind. It would take much effort and time on the part of clinicians and thoughtful psychological investigators to restore coherence and good practice in this vexed arena.

Although there is no evidence that the veterans of Vietnam were any more maladjusted than veterans of previous conflicts (indeed the tours of duty were specifically limited so as to avoid the prolonged exposures to battle stress of past wars), the PTSD diagnosis flourished in a charged political environment. The psychiatrists who promoted this new diagnosis were politically opposed to the war in Southeast Asia and deplored in particular the suffering of soldiers who had been drafted into that conflict.

Some of their patients were veterans who were having trouble adjusting to civilian life. Even pop culture—exemplified by the Martin Scorsese 1976 movie *Taxi Driver*—promoted the idea that the traumatic memories of service in Vietnam, both deeply buried and yet active in a distorted way in consciousness, commonly produced serious mental and behavioral disturbance in veterans.

Of course, many ex-military men and women felt few such aftereffects and went on to lead fruitful and satisfying civilian lives. But some veterans who, after discharge and for any number of reasons, failed in civilian life and fell into social instability, narcotics addiction, alcoholism, interpersonal hostility, and general unhappiness came to believe that they had been afflicted by some special mental condition brought on by their time in the war zone.

Because at first the veterans hospital system did not see these problems as "war wounds," given that they could represent the effects of personal characteristics that preceded military service, the believers in this new understanding of the psychological effects of warfare gathered in self-help groups to support the concept of a "post-Vietnam syndrome" and to spread the idea among other veterans.

Psychiatric advocates soon aligned themselves with these groups and maintained that the subjects' troublesome temperaments and aggressive behaviors came not from preexisting features of their makeup, but were the results of the warfare traumas to which they had been exposed and the "trauma memories" these experiences had produced. With PTSD, they were proposing a disease-like category generated by "trauma memories" that explained all the emotional and behavioral difficulties of the returning soldiers.

These advocates seized the opportunity to identify, codify, and affirm their ideas and to advance their propositions with some official diagnostic recognition. Working deliberately and effectively on the editorial committees of the American Psychiatric Association (APA), they were able in 1980 to get PTSD included in *DSM-III*.

Although initially suspicious of the diagnosis because of all the assumptions it carried, the Veterans Administration and its hospitals came to see how it provided the justification that every caregiving bureaucracy seeks for its services. Before long, the VA was devoting special units—almost entire hospitals—to PTSD cases.

The numbers of afflicted grew exponentially after the war. Some veterans hospitals, though, began to report fraudulent patients who claimed to have the symptoms associated with PTSD but were found never to have been in combat.[4] What now seems surprising is how long it took before critical thinking began in earnest.

In part this delay was the result of a concern that close examination of the PTSD concept might be—and often was—construed as a way of denying the suffering of soldiers and other distressed people. And so efforts to determine whether a diagnosis of PTSD adequately identified the problems many veterans faced was deplored even though correct diagnoses would have enhanced proper treatment. Some consequences of the careless acceptance of these diagnostic ideas became impossible to ignore.

For example, according to a study of Vietnam veterans released in 1988—the National Vietnam Veterans Readjustment Study (NVVRS)—as many as 479,000 of the 3.14 million men who had served in Vietnam still had PTSD, fifteen years after U.S. soldiers had left Southeast Asia. The commission also reported that almost 1 million veterans in all had had "full-blown" PTSD at some time—this, even though only 300,000 had ever been in combat. This was simply too much. Something obviously was wrong either in the conception of the problem or with its identification.

On reflection now, these numbers can be seen as the result of several problems with the way this survey identified PTSD cases. The diagnostic questionnaires cast a broad net, picking up many different kinds of distressed people and including them all under the diagnosis of PTSD. Most crucially, the survey did not access records to confirm the facts of battle or trauma claims. False and fraudulent claimants were swept up in the survey, but in unknown numbers.

Whatever the cause for these astonishing results, further studies of Vietnam veterans with PTSD diagnoses were launched. Results emerged that undercut claims that PTSD was common and that treatment directed at "traumatic memories" was what the veterans needed.

Among the most noteworthy was work by VA psychologists demonstrating that veterans in their hospitals with PTSD complaints tended to exaggerate their symptoms in psychometric studies—especially showing on psychological testing extreme elevations on the validity scales in a "fake bad" direction. These psychologists also began to check the claims of battle trauma in these patients and discovered that large numbers of them had few or no traumatic experiences documented in their service record. In fact, some of them had succeeded in gaining admission to the veterans hospital even though they had never been in the armed services.

More specific studies of the treatment programs themselves soon followed. A study of Vietnam veterans at the National Center for PTSD in West Haven, Connecticut, demonstrated that four months of intensive hospital care—including group therapy, individual therapy, behavioral therapy, family therapy, and vocational guidance focused on their memories and how these memories related to their symptoms and behaviors—actually made patients' psychiatric symptoms and family problems worse. There were also more suicide attempts, and no improvement in levels of substance abuse.

Israeli studies provide confirmation. These studies demonstrated that long-term hospital treatment of combat veterans that included a strong focus on encouraging the patients to "re-remember" and "draw up" their traumatic experiences and express the emotional feelings tied to them made their soldiers hypersensitive and worsened their symptoms. By encouraging the patients to concentrate on their psychological "wounds" in combat, the therapists kept them from solving individual here-and-now problems of adjustment postcombat, much to the detriment of recovery and rehabilitation. These examples dovetail with the original and simpler view of battle reactions as natural, grim, but self-limited responses.

The idea of "dissociated traumatic memories" has also encouraged the use of grief and disaster "counselors" at accident and disaster sites to prevent PTSD from emerging later in the witnesses and people directly involved in these incidents. Again, studies have not borne out the counselors' utility. Richard J. McNally led a 2003 investigation of debriefing by counselors after trauma and found that the practice had no diminishing effect on the overall rate of PTSD-like symptoms in survivors. In some cases, McNally found, it may increase the rate significantly by "consolidating" the emotional memories for continuing review and reflection.[5]

The new converts from MPD to PTSD added to its momentum. Figure 12.1 demonstrates that the PTSD craze went exponential in the 1990s, just as MPD began to fail. The enthusiasm for PTSD helped the advocates for "recovered" memories transform their MPD services into "trauma" services.

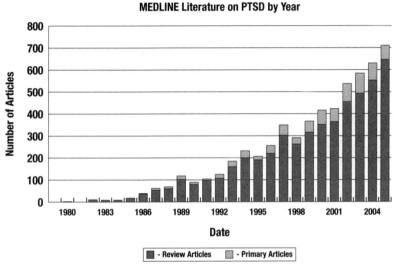

MEDLINE Literature on PTSD by Year

Figure 12.1. MEDLINE literature on PTSD by year. Results were derived from a MEDLINE search for English-language publications containing keywords "PTSD" or "post-traumatic stress disorder" for the years 1979–2005. (*Source:* Paul R. McHugh and Glenn Treisman, "PTSD: A Problematic Diagnostic Category," *Journal of Anxiety Disorders* 21 [2007]: 211–22. Used by permission.)

All the same colleagues—Judith Herman, Bessel van der Kolk, David Spiegel, Richard Loewenstein, and others—emerged center stage, once again talking about the need for "long-term psychotherapy," the "working through [of] traumatic memories," and even reintroducing "hypnosis [as] useful in teaching patients about the dissociative nature of their symptoms."[6]

Many studies of the diagnostic practices and therapeutic results for PTSD indicated that it was being overestimated and oversold. At the same time, other studies brought evidence that PTSD was not something distinct and different from other intense emotions of adjustment. It was not some kind of disease category, as many of its advocates had implied.

Thus many efforts were made to distinguish PTSD patients by some change in their body or brain. Enthusiasm came and went for "shrinkages" of strategic brain regions, such as the hippocampus; altered hormonal secretory patterns, particularly from the adrenal cortex; hyperactivity in limbic brain regions where emotions are aroused; and changes in physiologic functions, such as heart rate and skin conductance (the transmission of an electrical current through the skin following emotional sweat production). All proposed markers ultimately failed, either because they were not found on a regular basis with PTSD or were nonspecific in that they are found in many other examples of human emotional arousal—both normal and abnormal.

The Institute of Medicine attempted to resolve some of the debate over PTSD but unfortunately gave the task to a committee in which proponents of the idea that PTSD is a distinct and separate malady were overrepresented. Its report therefore works hard to prove that claim, but even so had to conclude that "no biomarkers are clinically useful or specific in diagnosing PTSD, assessing the risk of developing it, or charting its progression."[7]

And then there's the "Criterion A problem"—an amusing term for an issue that strikes at the heart of PTSD and its traumatic causation. This is an issue produced by the diagnostic method employed by *DSM-III/IV*.

For each psychiatric disorder, *DSM* lays out the features that the experts on that disorder describe as the criteria they use to identify cases of it. These criteria are listed successively (Criterion A, B, C, etc.) according to their significance and importance for the diagnosis of that disorder.

For PTSD, the criteria list in *DSM-IV* begins with Criterion A (stating essentially that the patient has been exposed to a serious and intensely distressing traumatic event) and Criteria B through D (the patient shows the mental symptoms generated by that experience). Using these criteria,

DSM-III/IV assumes that PTSD is a specific and categorically separate mental disorder produced by recognized traumas (Criterion A) and diagnostically identified by such symptoms as distress, anxiety, and wariness (Criteria B through D).

This seemed simple enough. The problem is that many patients show up complaining of the symptoms in Criteria B through D but report either no traumatic experiences or else events that do not rise to the level of "trauma," such as changing jobs, a fender bender, financial difficulties, or even hearing rumors of trouble. Hence the Criterion A problem. What to do?

A common way—and unfortunately one that possibly will get into *DSM-V*—is to extend the Criterion A conception to encompass all of life's troubles, including what might just be imagined, and claim that every one of them can produce PTSD. This has been called "criterion-creep" by McNally. But that way ultimately takes both the "P" for *post* and the "T" for *traumatic* out of PTSD, essentially purging it of significance.

To a clinician who holds PTSD to be an emotion of adjustment, the Criterion A problem presents no surprise. People simply differ in what they find disturbing—even "traumatic." Psychiatrists studying soldiers will emphasize the significance of dangerous events and perhaps deemphasize the contribution of the psychological traits of the individual when transforming an emotional reaction into a category of disorder. They did it during World War I with "shell shock."

Another PTSD issue is the so-called co-morbid problem. Patients who satisfy the diagnostic criteria for PTSD also satisfy the criteria for major depression, generalized anxiety disorder, panic disorder, and the like, especially when they are assessed using the standard "top-down" diagnostic screening instruments rather than the "bottom-up" approach. What to make of this problem?

Once again the pitfall is thinking of PTSD as a separate categorical condition. One has to be unlucky to have two distinct conditions at the same time—chicken pox and mumps—but one can have a response, even a very severe one, if it regularly accompanies a condition—nasty itching with chicken pox. Patients with panic anxiety have PTSD symptoms not because they are unlucky and have two maladies, but because panic anxiety presents the patient with many threatening challenges and thus provokes the emotion of adjustment.

What stands up now after all is said and done? How does any of it relate to searching for trauma—"trying to remember"—when asked to treat patients with mental disorders such as depression and anxiety? What should mental health professionals think and how should they practice?

They should begin with what exists and what we know. PTSD is a severe and persisting emotional response to life's challenges. It is not a mental disorder in any categorical sense, but a mental state that is noticed because of its intensity and duration rather than anything else "abnormal" about it.

All efforts to make it into a particular and distinct malady have failed. No biological mark differentiates patients with PTSD from normal emotionally distressed subjects, and many people have the very same state of mind and emotional symptoms without having suffered a traumatic experience.

Counting cases of PTSD (as did the National Vietnam Veterans Readjustment Study) will produce very different numbers in any population because what constitutes a case is so arbitrary. Much depends on how the investigators interpret the words *severe* and *persistent* when applied to an emotion or feeling. *No* independent, objective scales inform those interpretations. This arbitrary factor means that PTSD can be judged as so common that it afflicts all veterans or so rare as to be unusual even in survivors of ferocious battles.

Whatever decision is made about the prevalence of PTSD will be difficult to refute even though all may soon realize how it is affected by political, social, and institutional biases. For example, support for a war may lead to an emphasis on resilience and valor on the part of soldiers that encourages minimizing their emotional burdens, whereas rejection of a war may lead to an emphasis on injury and distress among soldiers that encourages exaggerating their emotional burdens.

More to the point, though, because the expressions of PTSD represent normal emotional responses to threat, they will be affected in both intensity and duration by a host of variables that include the severity or repetitiveness of the threats, the characteristics of the individual affected, and the social situations that surround both the events and the person. Specifically,

PTSD stands on three legs: the biology of human emotions (the features of the body and brain that generate and sustain intense feelings in response to events), the psychology of the subject (the cognitive and affective characteristics that bring resilience and vulnerability to individuals), and the social significance of the situation (the way the people involved interpret the provocative events). Each contributes crucially, and how this triad of influences is managed will determine the severity, persistence, and resolution of this emotion of adjustment.

None of this, however, is mysterious to any clinician who has helped patients with severe and long-lasting conditions such as persistent grief. With patients suffering from extreme grief, experienced doctors first identify any illness that may be confused with (or may have been precipitated by) grief and treat it. But, once they've excluded any other condition, these clinicians settle in to help the patient by discerning what has either sustained the grief or made it so severe. Exactly the same treatment should be given patients with persisting symptoms of PTSD.

A typical systematic approach begins by first learning about and considering details of the patient's life *prior to the trauma*, such as characteristics of personal development, previous mental illnesses, and habits. Then the psychiatrist reviews aspects of the patient *concurrent or coexisting with the trauma*, such as his or her age, sex, personality, social standing, and role in the events. Finally, the psychiatrist makes note of any issues of significance to the patient that have appeared *subsequent to the trauma*, such as social supports, emerging life challenges and opportunities, and any new and independent stresses.

By coming to know these matters thoroughly—matters of the here and now—the mystery of severe and persisting PTSD will disappear. The distress and difficulties arising from this emotion of adjustment, as with any other, are entirely manageable by competent psychotherapists who attend to matters of the present and future in ways that I shall discuss in the following chapters.

Information of this sort proves of little interest to those therapists drawn to the diagnosis of PTSD primarily so they can again search for and recover memories. The concept of traumatic memory is a red herring distracting the attention of these therapists. Not only is traumatic memory a clinically unnecessary concept, what exactly is "remembered" as the most distressing feature of an experience is often (as mentioned earlier) decided in retrospect, after the "fact," especially by therapists persuaded that something mysterious is in play.

Distressed feelings, nightmares, agitation, and the like are products with many different sources. They can accompany a wide variety of psychiatric disorders, and they accompany all of the emotions of adjustment. In fact, they will occur whenever distressing ideas are being generated. This explains why seeking to "recover" memories of childhood abuse will often evoke distressing emotional reactions in patients that then are often confused as PTSD responses to the memories themselves.

And so the burning question to ask of the trauma centers replacing the old "multiple personality centers" is whether they are inducing such emotional distress (and calling it PTSD) when seeking to "recover" trauma memories, just as previously they induced MPD when seeking to "recover" sexual abuse memories. Given that techniques such as hypnosis and suggestive probing of recall are still being employed, good reasons exist for asking that question.

13

Making Sense of Psychotherapy

The destructive impact of the recovered memory and traumatic memory concepts on the psychiatric profession does not derive primarily from the error rates of the practices associated with them—although the rates are high and the practices have led to the persecution of many innocent people, have provoked public chaos and controversies requiring courtroom intervention for settlement, and continue to confuse us over the psychological status of war veterans. Neither does it depend on any sense that the crimes and traumas reported in therapy are implausible in themselves. No one is denying that child abuse happens and can be hidden by its perpetrators, or that people can fail to remember all the details of a traumatic event. And certainly everyone agrees that battlefield experiences can shake even the most valiant and that terrors can have long-lasting psychological effects.

What has rendered these concepts so destructive to psychiatric practice is that they have become for their advocates, not possibilities to be considered among others when diagnosing patients, but causal preconceptions carried with the force of fervent convictions into their practice. This is what makes these advocates so ready to abuse their authority and attack their challengers.

Although any preconception will drive errors into medical or psychological treatment, these particular biases—carried with such emotional conviction, advanced with such vehemence, and defended despite powerful counterevidence—have drawn psychotherapists along fixed and rigid paths and blinded them (and eventually their patients) to alternative explanations.

Their passionate convictions—that they are rooting out villains and helping victims of misused power—draw these therapists away from their responsibility for establishing the empirical truth of the clinical situation before they launch therapy. It explains why they fail to employ modes of assessment that reduce error (such as finding and consulting with external informants) and why they never think it crucial to assess the accuracy of "recovered" memories (by, for example, employing the 2 × 2 table). As William Butler Yeats notes in "The Second Coming" (1921): "Things fall apart ... / ... [when] the worst / Are full of passionate intensity."[1]

As I've emphasized throughout this book, psychotherapy resting on convictions and suspicious preconceptions has been the bane of psychiatry since Sigmund Freud. The Mannerists of today, whether they are pressing the concepts of multiple personality disorder or post-traumatic stress disorder, are responsible for the increased levels of distrust in psychotherapy among the general public.

Paradoxically enough, at the very time these "memory workers" were misleading both their professional colleagues and their patients with fundamentally flawed concepts and practices, a sound and clarifying set of ideas about the nature of psychotherapy and how to work best with patients was gaining ground within psychiatry and impressing those committed to a responsible form of practice. In this chapter and the next, I will describe this work and how, despite its value and importance, the concepts emerging from it have been—and essentially still are—ignored by those who continue to adhere to their misguided notions about memory.

Psychotherapy, like any other form of treatment, can do harm. It is now possible to identify the attributes of psychotherapy that, if misemployed or misunderstood, can transform it from a beneficial practice into a vehicle for false memories and false assumptions—and so explain how it could, in the hands of some practitioners, lead thousands falsely to accuse their parents of the grossest and vilest acts or render shaken soldiers and victims of violence invalids by insisting that they dwell on and embellish their past experiences.

One makes sense of psychotherapy as a practice—and thus becomes armed against its misuse—in three ways: first, by identifying it as a mode of care; second, by distinguishing two distinct families of psychotherapies with important and practical differences; and third, by describing how an optimal form of psychotherapy came to be discerned and put into practice essentially at the same time the Manneristic Freudians were inflicting their cruel injuries on patients and families.

I believe this information will certainly help those who are considering undergoing psychotherapy but who, if they have heard about these injuries, worry about the risks involved. More generally, I am confident that anyone interested in the quality of mental health care as a whole will now want answers to such questions as: What should patients expect in psychotherapy? Have some forms of psychotherapy proved safer than others and why? and How might patients already in psychotherapy decide whether they are being properly treated?

I wish to emphasize at the outset that much of the information about psychotherapy that I provide in this and the following chapter was available to therapists and patients before the false memory craze began. Just as Martin Orne had identified the uses and abuses of hypnosis, just as textbook teaching had identified multiple personality disorder as a form of hysteria, and just as Elizabeth Loftus had identified how human memory is vulnerable to suggestion, so psychologists and psychiatrists such as Kurt Lewin, Jerome Frank, and Aaron T. Beck had described the basic nature of psychotherapy and proffered approaches that avoid errors and benefit patients.

However, prior to the false memory craze, psychotherapy was viewed too uncritically and always as benign. Many in the public, if familiar only with Hollywood depictions of therapists or informed only by literary scholars telling them that new knowledge about human nature was emerging, came to think of psychotherapy as a rite or ritual, a secular ritual to be sure but, like any ritual, a mysterious and fascinating phenomenon beyond their capacity to scrutinize and judge.

What we in the profession can teach now—and perhaps emphasize more in light of the disastrous consequences of the repressed memory movement—is that psychotherapy, like any treatment, can injure as much as it can help. At the same time, there is nothing magical or mysterious about it. Psychotherapy is a mode of addressing human mental problems and distress, a mode that in some form or other is found in every culture. To properly understand it, one should not be distracted by the many and diverse theories generated by its practitioners, but should direct attention toward therapists' manifest actions. When one looks at what therapists actually strive to do and how they do it, the benefits and hazards in psychotherapy become obvious.

I'll start by addressing a central source of confusion. Although the term *psychotherapy* evokes notions of medical or surgical procedures, the methods employed in its practice are fundamentally different from them. Medical and surgical procedures aim to cure a disrupted body by removing or repairing structural or functional pathologies. Gains and losses—both temporary and permanent—accompany these procedures, but they can be prudently acknowledged, directly assessed, and dispassionately weighed against one another—and also against no treatment—in light of what doctors already know about how diseases advance and injuries impair.

Psychotherapy does not aim to cure the body—or the brain, for that matter; it aims to sway the mind. It is a persuasive process—a way of influencing a person to think and behave differently. The gains and losses induced by its influence can range from the benefits of enhanced self-control and social flourishing to the injuries of coercive misdirection and vicious seduction.

Patients in psychotherapy—like all patients, given that they are distressed and seeking assistance from those they presume to be experts—are vulnerable to exploitation. But in psychotherapy, where persuasion is the essence of the treatment, patients may feel, for at least some time, that they must be less critical and more trusting of the process. This is a mistake that rests to some extent on the diffidence of the uninformed.

Even if we put the inventions about memory to one side, anyone considering psychotherapy should ask such questions as: Do I really need psychological influence or can I resolve these matters myself? Who might be best at helping me? How will any influence on my thoughts and actions be exerted? What will be expected of me? What clear goals of treatment do I have? What are the possible complications of this treatment? How might I decide whether I've improved?

Psychotherapy has so insinuated itself into our culture that patients seldom ask these questions of their therapists, and therapists seldom anticipate and address them with the patients before launching into treatment. In many circles, such questions can seem as deeply impertinent as inquiring about the merit of schooling in our lives. Such blind trust permitted the false memory craze to get a head start. Following are several points anyone considering psychotherapy should reflect upon.

First, understand what psychotherapy cannot do. As the treatment rests upon talk, it cannot "cure" a disease of the brain that disables its mental faculties or powers. Psychotherapy can play a helpful, even enhancing, role in rehabilitation from such a disease, however, and can amplify considerably the effects of medication by sustaining compliance and directing the patients into hopeful ways of thinking. But talk alone will not cure any disruption of mental faculties that rests upon disease or defect. Doctors need to address the issues with physical measures, such as medications.

Second, psychotherapy will not change innate or constitutional psychological features. It cannot add a single point to someone's IQ, transform an extravert into an introvert, or vice versa. But psychotherapists certainly can help people recognize the assets and vulnerabilities they derive from their natures and use this information to guide them toward aspirations, activities, or paths in life where they can be successful and flourish. In particular, psychotherapy can address and help correct awkward, unhelpful attitudes and assumptions that come more easily to those with certain temperaments—such as the pessimism of introverts that can lead them into self-defeating lines of behavior. Constructive psychotherapy can help patients choose educational programs and ways of life that fit with their intellectual powers and strengthen their skills.

Third, a sizable proportion of patients, as many as two out of three, who are referred for psychotherapy because of anxiety or depressive symptoms would, if left alone, spontaneously recover—although the recovery may be by most standards rather slow and take months or even a few years to occur. This fact of spontaneous remission from states of mind that are so often the focus of psychotherapy came to light in several ways.

The first revealing contribution came from two teachers of mine, Michael Shepherd and Ernest Gruenberg, who estimated the duration of such illnesses by employing a simple and standard rule of epidemiology. This rule holds that the "prevalence [P] of a condition in a population at a designated time (i.e. the total number of cases with the condition) is the product of the incidence [I]of the condition over time (i.e. the number of new cases falling ill with the condition) and its duration [D]." That is, $P = I \times D$.

Because they had good data on both the incidence and prevalence of anxious and depressive states in the New York population from the Health Insurance Plan of Greater New York, Shepherd and Gruenberg could solve for the average duration of these conditions. They determined that although these distressful states of mind may be of long duration in some people and of short duration in others, "the best available data would suggest an average duration between one and two years."[2]

Spontaneous recovery from these states should not come as a big surprise. As far back as the nineteenth century, with the beginnings of psychiatric care, many hospitals reported that the majority of their patients recovered when given the "moral therapy" of the day. But given spontaneous recovery, investigators striving to study and then prescribe any treatment for psychiatric patients—with medications, group therapy, individual psychotherapy—must demonstrate that the treatment either speeds this process of natural recovery or helps those patients who would not otherwise improve. Demonstrating both faster recoveries and recovery of the more recalcitrant 30 percent or so of patients (the typical and not inconsiderable minority in anxious and depressive disorders, after all) must be the test. Obviously, to make such a demonstration the treatment group must be compared in their recovery rates and numbers against some kind of untreated control group of patients.

Fourth, the good news is that several investigators, understanding how they had to demonstrate that treatments improved on spontaneous recovery, successfully developed new and better psychotherapeutic procedures in the 1970s. They did so usually by challenging the Freudian therapies that were at the time dominant.

The most persistent and forceful challenger to the claims of Freudian psychotherapy was the German-born British psychologist Hans Eysenck, who held that its claims were unsupported by anything solid, such as patient comparisons and follow-ups. Likewise, in the United States the investigative work of Jerome Frank at Hopkins and Aaron T. Beck of the University of Pennsylvania illuminated the problems tied to contemporary claims for psychotherapy.

Much mutual interest developed between Hopkins and the University of Pennsylvania as psychotherapy was closely studied and ultimately changed for the better. Therapy was better understood and particular practices were identified as clear improvements over those of the past.

Both Frank and Beck were broadly experienced psychiatrists knowledgeable in most forms of psychotherapy. Both had early in their studies undergone a personal Freudian psychoanalysis. But both worked closely with critical psychological scientists and brought to the study of patients an empirical stance—and that move ultimately drove the mystery from psychotherapy and led to the development of the better programs we have today.

In this chapter, I shall concentrate on Jerome Frank's work on psychotherapy done at Johns Hopkins from the late 1950s through the 1980s. His aim was not so much to produce a new kind of psychotherapy as to reveal what psychotherapy is and what patients can get from it. In the next chapter, I shall concentrate on Aaron T. Beck's work in devising a new psychotherapy that provided exactly what Frank had seen as optimal.

Frank was a first-rate investigator and psychiatrist. His interests in psychological matters derived from his early education with the German psychologist Kurt Lewin, who held—in contrast to Freud—that most people's emotional and behavioral problems related to their current life circumstances or situations and how they were responding to them. Lewin believed that the childhood or early life of patients was relevant in that any human life is a continuum and events in childhood can bias a person's assumptions, but he further believed that this shaping was seldom if ever the most pressing factor explaining their current state of mind. And he also held that addressing these background matters would not lead to prompt resolution of the symptoms presented by the patient.

Lewin's emphasis on the importance of the here and now in therapy provoked in Frank reservations about the traditional Freudian emphasis on the role of abiding unconscious conflicts derived from childhood as the root cause of mental disorders. Frank planned to confirm or refute Lewin by studying patients who were being treated in the psychotherapy clinics at Hopkins.

Frank's methods of assessing patients were broad-ranging and included thorough examinations of their past histories and present situations. He studied therapies that succeeded and therapies that failed. He drew in many associates with excellent scientific and clinical credentials who helped assess the patients and think about research directions.

Frank and his group soon realized that much of what was claimed for psychotherapy depended on stories or anecdotes about prototypic patients. Freud's classic case descriptions (Dora, Little Hans, Wolf Man, etc.) were, with better historical reporting, now seen as forced interpretations and misrepresentations of facts. Peter Kramer dubbed them "Freud's train wrecks."[3]

Frank decided that he and his group should begin again and look at the clinical conditions of patients who sought psychotherapeutic help to see what they had in common and what changes seemed to occur in them if they improved. He and his colleagues gathered information from hundreds of patients, diverse in background and in symptoms, and thus could confidently derive several important general principles about people who seek psychotherapy and about the process of psychotherapy itself—at least the kind offered at Hopkins.

What Frank found in his close study of patients was that, just as Lewin thought, many different factors in their contemporary life circumstances provoked their distress. This could be discerned even though the patients' therapists often believed in the Freudian theory and were actively striving to make their patients fit their preconceptions.

In essence, the patients had many different provocations for their problems, and contrary to what Freud had taught, it was impossible to transform these provocations into expressions of intangible unconscious conflict. For all that the patients were different in regard to the causes of their distresses, they were remarkably similar in how they expressed the problems for which they were seeking help from the clinic. These patients resembled one another in the distress they presented, not in what caused it.

Frank demonstrated that the patients seeking psychotherapy all displayed some mixture of anxiety and depression, sometimes tinged with resentment and often accompanied by a sense of alienation from others, such as family and friends. They were disheartened by some aspects of life's challenges and were struggling to overcome what they faced. They tended to be pessimistic, despairing that they would be able to regain their self-control and equilibrium. This despair, as much as the symptoms themselves, prompted them to seek psychotherapeutic assistance.

Frank, on recognizing how similarities in their suffering rather than in its cause characterized these patients, defined their disheartened discouragement and anxiety as "demoralization." He thought of this state as a kind of endpoint reached by patients driven by any number of provocations. Those might include mental illnesses, temperaments conducive to helplessness or hopelessness in the face of adversity, and self-defeating but habitual assumptions that they had taken up earlier in life.

Frank concluded that the patients had sought psychotherapy for the same reasons that people had traditionally turned to those they presumed wiser or more expert in dealing with life's problems and from whom they sought reassurance, hope, and support. People were willing to believe that psychotherapists could provide this help, just as in the past they believed they could find it from priests, rabbis, and ministers of God.

In characterizing their plight in this way, Frank taught that psychotherapy patients were "overmastered" by their life circumstances, and he demonstrated how this sense of loss of mastery had generated their demoralization.

He saw psychotherapy as endeavoring to advance persuasive ideas on how to better manage life circumstances and choices. Frank held that the main effort of psychotherapists—whether they realized it or not—was to help patients regain some understanding of just how they had been overcome and what it would take to regain their sense of mastery over life's challenges and presenting situations.

Frank did not fail to search for all sources of the demoralized state. He was quite willing to believe that in a given patient it may have been some mental illness, such as major depression, that would need medication for its relief, or that it may have been some particular situation—even one susceptible to a Freudian interpretation.

He simply emphasized the importance of recognizing the patient's individuality in this matter and appreciating just how out of control he or she had come to feel. Whatever one does in psychotherapy, he taught—and by means of any combination of psychotherapy, medications, and guidance—be sure to perceive the individual's situation and thus discern how the demoralized condition is understandable.

Frank noted, though, that a therapeutic program that might persuade and restore one group of patients might not prove helpful to another. Hence, he explained, the different schools of psychotherapists (i.e., Freudian, Adlerian, Jungian, Rogerian, etc.), each of which believed it was uniquely insightful and qualified, each of which found patients who responded to its particular position, but every one of which was doing something similar: suggesting to patients a way of mastering life circumstances and finding some who accepted and others who rejected its point of view.

Perhaps the most crucial fact that Frank revealed was that a successful treatment does not depend on whether the suggestions the patients follow are better, truer, or more scientifically established than any others. What seemed to heal the patients in his study was whatever they found most persuasive, not what could be proven factually true with them.

From what he saw, he could not identify a royal road to relieving demoralization. Different patients found relief from different—even contrary—therapeutic programs. He emphasized this point when he noted how traditional "healers" in the past or in other cultures were apparently capable of generating similar recoveries from demoralization with ideas and practices that would never be accepted today.

Frank's research into psychotherapy ultimately helped many psychiatrists committed to empirical work abandon the Freudian idea that the cause of mental distress comes from some universal conflict fundamental to human development and generated in early life through the interactions of the selfish infant and the socializing forces of the family. Most patients are demoralized, as Lewin taught, by what they are confronting in the present. Habits of thought derived from their past and from aspects of their psychological constitution can amplify their problems and retard their solutions, but those factors are less important than the proximate contemporary challenges they face.

Just as Frank demonstrated that a variety of psychotherapeutic practices could help some patients "master" their situations and regain their "morale," he also could explain why many patients with identical symptoms and situations recovered spontaneously. They had found some way of their own to master their challenging situations—probably helped by fortunate combinations of strengths in their character, improved life circumstances, and advice from teachers, ministers, friends, and relatives.

Although Frank could not demonstrate that therapists committed to any particular theory or school of psychotherapy were more effective than any others with demoralized patients, he did note three characteristics common to all therapies. He came to believe that it was these general features of the therapeutic procedure—displayed in various ways and given different salience from one therapeutic school to another—rather than the particular theories driving the practices that helped patients recover. Again he noted that traditional "healers" shared these characteristics in their practices.

First, effective psychotherapists emphasize and display certain attributes of status in their behavioral style, dress, and titles that help patients view them as having the power and authority to heal them. Such accoutrements as wearing white coats, displaying diplomas on the office wall, and carrying the title "doctor" or "professor" play a part in generating necessary trust and confidence in the authority of the therapist and the psychotherapy program he or she prescribes.

Second, effective psychotherapy usually includes some effort at promoting some emotional arousal in the patients. These efforts may take the subtle form of evoking hope in a better future, a comforting sense that help will be available even if matters worsen, or a feeling of devotion and trust (occasionally to the point of adulation) for the therapist. He noted how in some therapies the therapist generates emotional states of a more purposeful and focused kind by drawing the patient's attention either to the dramatic aspects of the demoralizing problems that brought them to treatment or to the growing emotional ties between the patient and the therapist.

Third, effective therapists eventually offer their patients suggestions for action or for responding to circumstances. In some forms of therapy, these suggestions may arise subtly in the course of the interactions between the therapist and the patient, but in others they may come from the therapist in much the same way a physician might prescribe a medication. The suggestions—however delivered—encourage the patients to act upon and alter their situations and so begin to gain at least some feeling of control over their circumstances and take the first steps toward "mastery."

Further work between a therapist and a patient may involve refining actions, developing better plans, and emphasizing aspects of the results and their implications. Such work will continue to enhance patients' confidence that the therapy will bring them success in the matters that have demoralized them.

All effective psychotherapies use these three elements in one way or another, differing only in emphasis. For example, some therapists claim that helping patients reflect on the therapeutic relationship brings about the actions needed to promote healing and mastery by encouraging them to see the similarity between that relationship and other interactions in their lives. Other therapists propose that emotional arousal teaches their patients that they can survive the worst of their fears and with that reassurance they can move forward more actively. Still others hold that through prompting behavior they emphasize how recovery is fundamentally dependent on overcoming inertia, habits of thought, and conditioned fears. Frank would say that these are but distinctions in emphasis from among the three commonalities: (1) healer status, (2) emotional arousal, and (3) directions of action.

It was through studying patients over time and noting their responses that Frank came to realize and eventually emphasize—especially as he noted the central role of persuasion in psychotherapy—that these three themes appear in all modes of human interpersonal influence and the development of convictions. Persuasions of this sort are certainly not restricted to psychotherapy. They have been studied and shown to be remarkably powerful in laboratory settings, and they can be recognized in various forms of social propaganda and group activities that have sometimes gone wildly awry, with the most damaging of results.

Status (lab-coated authorities, official-looking machinery), emotions (increasing tensions that confuse and alter one's sense of situation), and directives (instructions to move ahead) were all in play in the remarkable and revealing experiments of the Yale social psychologist Stanley Milgram, who in the 1960s demonstrated that ordinary people could be persuaded—under the guise of participating in a scientific experiment—to give what they were told were dangerous shocks to protesting subjects (there were actually no shocks, and the subjects were collaborators with the investigators). Amazing to all (including the investigators) was that the majority of ordinary people, many of whom had advanced educations and social responsibilities, would persist in what they were convinced was painful, cruel, and dangerous treatment of other people.

They persisted in their actions because they were being told by a figure of authority that they had to remain a "part of an important experiment" and continue to follow the instructions in using punishment to "improve" how humans learn. This "scientific" story and the others' presumed place in it were sufficient to persuade the participants to continue their actions and abandon their natural sense of fellow feeling for suffering people or any duty to protect them.

With similar methods of persuasion, but cast not in terms of secular science backed up by evoked feelings of "responsibility" but in terms of religious authority backed up by evoked feelings of persecution and dependence, Jim Jones persuaded 910 of his followers in Jonestown, Guyana, to drink a cyanide-laced Kool-Aid-like beverage en masse and die together in a methodical, obedient, and public fashion. Essentially no one protested or failed to follow the leader's direction, even as they witnessed the painful deaths of their coreligionists.

These events reveal just how difficult it can be to say no to an "authority." And this is certainly true of demoralized patients seeking help from psychotherapists, as Frank taught. What happened in the false memory craze was that psychotherapists used their persuasive authority and the vulnerability of patients seeking support and hope to draw those patients into a willing form of self-deception about reality. The patients accepted the therapists' claims about sexual trauma and repression and were ultimately convinced that they had forgotten memories of the most astonishing kind and needed a great deal of help—in the form of tranquilizing medications, group inductions, and hypnotic trances—to "regain" these memories.

Some patients returned to their families and abandoned their false memories when for one reason or another they separated from their recovered memory therapists. I've mentioned how Donna Smith recovered her coherence and abandoned her false memories when she was sent from Maryland, where she had been under the influence of her therapists, to foster parents in Michigan, where she was free from that influence. But not all false memory patients recovered their coherence, and many to this day believe the stories that were imposed on them.

I mentioned in Chapter 12 how the psychotherapists focusing on "traumatic memories" in VA services for PTSD succeeded only in worsening their patients' psychiatric symptoms and behaviors. The therapies were misdirected, and the patients were injured.

Students of influence who teach that authority carries formidable power suggest that two approaches help in avoiding inappropriate influence or overcoming it when it is being exerted. These are worth noting.

The first way to fight influence is simply to decide whether the authority you are being asked to accept is actually an expert in the matter at hand. Many patients who fell into a false memory were being treated by therapists whose credentials were modest (some with music or education degrees) and whose knowledge about psychotherapy was acquired through so-called continuing education programs on recovered memory therapy. Such therapists, numerous though they are, should always be avoided for any course of serious psychological treatment.

The second method for resisting influence—even with someone who has expert credentials—is to ask yourself whether the expert is gaining something from your compliance. Do these experts have some financial gain tied to the enterprise, such as building an institution, a church, or a following around their beliefs? Do they seem pressured by other circumstances— fiscal, institutional, legal, and the like—to promote their ideas? Do they mention these commitments if you show some resistance? Do they tend to make the situation one in which it's "us against the world?" Do they fail to encourage feedback about the therapy, its implications, and its effects? The psychotherapeutic "experts" who generated the disasters of recovered memory had many of these characteristics—as revealed often in court statements and close scrutiny of clinic records.

Any person contemplating psychotherapy needs to see it as a form of influence and so choose a therapist carefully. In the next chapter, I will delve into how therapies can be distinguished from one another and explore the kind of therapy that has emerged that is most worthy of a patient's investment in time, money, and trust.

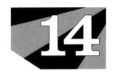

The "Conflict"
and the "Deficit"
Psychotherapies

A glance at the telephone directory's Yellow Pages reveals the huge marketplace built around psychotherapy today. Nurses, social workers, psychologists, educationalists, and counselors of many stripes far outnumber psychiatrists. They all advertise their readiness and assertively declare their suitability to provide psychotherapeutic services. How does anyone, especially one in need, navigate this marketplace and find the best help? What important differences exist in the way therapists conduct their treatments? Can patients anticipate how they will be treated given the therapists they choose? What kind of practice should they spurn? I hear such questions often, and in answering them I've relied on a useful division of psychotherapists separate from their professional qualifications.

Although all work by persuasion, they can be subdivided into two large families, distinguished by their view of the nature of the psychological problems that produce the demoralized, overmastered condition that brings patients to them. One group strives to identify some psychological conflict as the source of psychological unrest, and the other strives to grasp how some deficit in understanding has led to and sustains their difficulties.

The "conflict" family has been dominant since Freud, but the "deficit" family is now ascendant and proving itself. Both, though, need to be understood, as these fundamental distinctions between the two groups determine just how they think about the problems and treat their patients.

The conflict family, as mentioned, has been the dominant psychotherapy group since Freud and is the one to which the recovered memory therapists and the "traumatologists" naturally belong. All psychotherapists of this persuasion assume that some underlying, usually unconscious, conflict over life's demands is interfering with their patients' psychological capacities and has produced their demoralized condition. This conflict needs to be brought into the light of consciousness to be resolved.

Many psychiatrists and psychologists find themselves drawn to this conflict model of psychotherapy. They tend to explain their choice when questioned by saying that they believe such an approach not only will be a way of helping patients but also will benefit them personally by revealing much about the mysteries of human existence and development. Of course, they believe these alluring secrets are known only to an elite group.

Such workers usually speak of the conflict model of psychotherapy as a "modern" approach, one deep in its conceptions of the human mind and having a true sense of the human predicament, where natural affection, hierarchies of authority, and the demands of society evoke conflict and distress. They especially emphasize that in their treatments they tear away the masks or veils hiding the dismaying truths that are the real causes of human mental distress. They see patients as unwitting victims either of a punitive and coercive culture or, specifically, of a violent and exploitative parental figure and family structure. These therapists hold that their task is to discover the ways abusive power has injured their patients, to bring those facts into the light of awareness, and, when appropriate, to call to account the agents of that abuse.

They tend to suggest points of view to their subjects such as: "Things are not what they seem. Don't take your feelings of devotion to parents and happy memories of childhood at face value. See that what is upsetting you may well derive from experiences and family attitudes that at the moment are hidden from your consciousness." This "unmasking" impulse was at the heart of the recovered memory work. Freudian psychoanalysis provided the historic foundation for this impulse and encouraged it by its hermeneutics of suspicion.

These therapies tend to be long-term and self-perpetuating as more and more of the nature and contexts of "conflicts" are developed in therapy and call for "resolution." (Remember Patty Burgus and her years of treatment in Chicago and the eighteen months of in-patient treatment imposed on Donna Smith.) The idea that they are the victims of some mistreatment—from parents, the Vietnam War, civilization itself—often makes these patients slow to develop ownership of their own mental well-being. This keeps them dependent on psychological assistance and in long-term therapy.

Owing to the Freudian concept and mystique, therapists committed to the conflict forms of psychotherapy are often inattentive to the role induction aspects of their therapy. Indeed, they may display little openness to their patients about the role of persuasion in the treatment and emphasize the "enlightening" or even "astonishing" potential built into their psychotherapeutic efforts. They may introduce their enterprise to the patient as one of exploration, with analogies to open-ended laboratory studies and with expectations of "discoveries yet to come" as to the cause of the patient's distress.

Most conflict-directed therapists may mention that a close relationship will develop between the patient and the therapist. They expect the emotional aspects of this relationship to illuminate—even "reproduce"—vital features of patients' ways of dealing with parents and others in their life and so identify how habits of thought hinder their ability to flourish as adults. In this way, they hope to help their patients develop more positive ways of thinking and responding to conflict. I've seen patients who have done well with this form of therapy, but usually they were individuals who could cooperate with the therapy and still retain a grasp on their own reality that protected them from becoming overly dependent or credulous.

The other group of therapists works on the assumption that some deficits in psychological skills or some mistaken attitudes—either a kind of cognitive maladjustment or some overlearned emotional response style—lie behind their patients' demoralized, overmastered condition. They work at identifying the harmful consequences of thinking and responding in these ways and suggest better modes of thought and behavior. The psychotherapies that fall into this group include the twelve-step program practiced by Alcoholics Anonymous (AA), family therapy directed at improved practice of family roles and responsibilities, various forms of behavioral treatments directed at extinguishing phobias and obsessions, and, most especially, cognitive behavioral therapy (CBT).

For many physicians, the view that clinical problems derive from deficits or functional flaws is congenial. It matches how they customarily think when doing physical rehabilitative work, and thus they see their influence over patients in deficit-directed psychotherapy as yet another way of helping people recover themselves.

They find nothing incompatible with medical practice when they make such corrective suggestions to their patients as "You're not so strong in this area; we will explore ways by which you can strengthen yourself," or (directly from the AA manual) "You're powerless against alcohol and it has made your life unmanageable; [the key for regaining your future is not drinking]," or "Let's see if by confronting your fear of flying you can overcome your avoidance of it," or "The ideas that come to you in these situations are bound to produce feelings of misery and hopelessness—why not try thinking about them in another, perhaps more effective way and practice putting yourself in similar situations but with other people who count in your life?"

This form of treatment, with its prototype cognitive behavioral therapy, is by its nature goal-directed. It is intentionally tied to the patient's symptoms and own sense of what's lost or missing and what needs to be restored. This treatment usually demonstrates in a direct fashion just how demoralized feelings are products of maladaptive assumptions, false images of the world, and behavioral reflexes that need to be challenged and replaced if one hopes to regain and sustain a sense of mastery and control of one's life. And, perhaps most crucially, it emphasizes how much mental health and happiness is one's own responsibility.

This therapy tends to be relatively brief—ten to fifteen weekly sessions rather than years of treatment demanded by the long-term conflict therapies launched by Freudian psychoanalysis and copied by the recovered memory and trauma memory therapists.

Although CBT is a program of treatment that certainly can be repeated if the patient relapses, it aims to provide long-term skills. By its nature—emphasizing assessment and the role of self-direction—this therapy approximates some of the ways patients who have spontaneously recovered describe the course they followed.

In fact, the leaders of CBT (and some of the behavioral treatment programs that preceded it) right from the start compared their results with patients against those with untreated control patients so as to demonstrate that their treatments brought psychological improvement more swiftly and more regularly. Aaron T. Beck (known to all his friends and colleagues as Tim) emphasized the importance of such comparisons and what they revealed about the recovery of mental balance and self-mastery. In his very first book on depression (now a classic in CBT), he could point out how identifying and promptly challenging the maladaptive, depression-generating thoughts and images of his patients helped them.

One of Tim Beck's critical concepts was that therapists don't so much "cure" their patients as they "collaborate" with them in the search for better ways of thinking and responding to the situations in which they are living. His concept expands on the view that CBT works in ways similar to those that bring about spontaneous recoveries. But it certainly hastens the process and makes explicit what patients should learn from their recovery so as to sustain it.

These distinctions in the basic assumptions between the conflict psychotherapies, which deal with "memories," and the deficit psychotherapies, which deal with "cognitions and behavior," are at the heart of strenuous debates over psychotherapy today. Feelings and loyalties run high, because much about what constitutes the reality of human mental life and its travails is at stake.

One significant difference worth noting is that the deficit therapies—in particular, CBT—by successfully demonstrating their benefits in therapeutic trials against results seen for control patients have brought CBT strong support from critical observers. Clinicians with a practical bent have increasingly turned to it.

Yet both kinds of psychotherapy are forms of influence. With CBT, however, patients entering into treatment essentially establish a contract explaining how the treatment will be carried out and what it demands from both the patient and the therapist. Immediately after evaluating the patient, the CBT therapist strives to explain just how the therapy will proceed and why the therapist believes it will help. These efforts defuse any mystery that the patients may have brought with them to therapy. They encourage the patient to ask any question—simple or complex—about what to expect.

CBT is not bashful about its direct approach. From the very beginning, the therapist makes clear that the treatment is a matter of persuasion directed at helping the patient understand how to recover. It identifies that effort at persuasion as emerging from a joint effort to understand the life circumstances and challenges the patient faces and to characterize the patient's habits of thought and feelings in those situations.

The CBT therapist flatly asserts, and thus does much to reassure the patient, that these habits and responses are not too difficult to address and that clinical experience with other patients has demonstrated how, with their modification, recovery from states of depression and anxiety can be expected.

CBT therapists will specifically describe to their patients (1) how they will be asked to identify particular situations where they have felt overmastered and distressed, (2) how the therapists will work with them to discern thoughts, attitudes, and images provoked in and by those situations, and (3) how the therapists will help them find other ways to think, imagine, and respond in these and similar situations so that (4) a means of preventing emotional distress and the accompanying sense of being out of control and overmastered will be explicitly identified, studied, and practiced.

While some CBT therapists may speak of this important introductory phase of treatment as that of "contracting," there are other ways of describing what they do as they set up the therapeutic plan. Martin Orne referred to this stage as "anticipatory socialization," and Jerome Frank referred to it as "role induction"—both appreciating just how crucial this introductory phase was in all forms of psychotherapy.

Orne emphasized that therapists should not assume that patients understand anything about psychotherapy. Indeed, he taught that one should assume that patients have all sorts of confused—even weird—ideas about the process and that only a clear set of statements on launching the therapy—repeated whenever necessary during its course—as to the expectations, assumptions, and modes of procedure could help patients become truly informed subjects and coherent participants in the process.

Most CBT therapists end each weekly session by asking the patient for feedback. The therapist specifically asks the patient what, from his or her point of view, went well and what may have been either hard to understand or onerous to contemplate in that session. Not only does this feedback help demonstrate the therapist's concern for the patient and the process, but it keeps the collaborative nature of CBT in the forefront of everyone's thinking. No one is "the master;" both are working to make sense of circumstances and to find a way of responding that can relieve the feelings of demoralization that accompany them.

Given that psychotherapy is a persuasive way of reframing one's attitudes and assumptions, people should think seriously about what aspect of their lives they would be willing to see affected by another's influence before trying it. It's different from deciding to undergo a hip replacement after some years of painful disability. Both the decision to enter into psychotherapy and the choice of a psychotherapist are matters of moment. One is, after all, proposing to surrender some personal sovereignty in the hopes of advancing in understanding and gaining in skill.

For these reasons, psychotherapy should not be considered, as it is in some quarters, a rite of passage that everyone should undergo. I fear that in some cities young people are encouraged to think that the issues that represent their "coming of age"—those decisions about their convictions, commitments, and allegiances that bring with them a maturity and personal authenticity—are well and usefully addressed through an exploratory psychotherapy, usually one focused on confronting some inner conflict.

Young people thinking that way, most of them women, were the main prey of the recovered memory therapists. Perhaps they were overly sensitive to their feelings and uncertain about their future when they surrendered to these therapists' promises of insight and understanding.

What many of them were seeking in therapy they probably would have discerned naturally by trusting in what they would learn as they matured. Instead, by choosing to enter conflict psychotherapy, they found themselves much worse off than when they began. They became entangled in conflicts they'd never imagined, and as a result found themselves even more estranged from parents, siblings, spouses, and friends. And, in a dismaying number of cases, they were led into committing perjuries against innocent parents and others.

Psychotherapy is a serious and potentially disruptive process to be entered into only after careful consideration of the nature of the problems to be addressed. One should certainly ask oneself—and, if uncertain, a psychiatrist—whether the problems might well resolve themselves without addressing them in such a challenging way.

For all these reasons, psychotherapy should be "prescribed," not "tried out" as though it were some exercise routine. Its prescription should come from a psychiatrist and rest upon a thorough psychiatric assessment—an assessment that can define the problems, identify the goals of therapy, and provide an estimate of the cost of therapy in both time and money.

I emphatically hold that anyone thinking of psychotherapy should start by consulting a psychiatrist. Only through such a consultation and with a careful consideration of the modes of treatment presented should one decide to enter psychotherapy.

The psychotherapy should be provided either by the psychiatrist consulted or by a therapist the psychiatrist can recommend on the basis of his or her past experience with that therapist. And, if the psychiatrist is not providing the therapy, then he or she should be willing to check the patient's progress over time and regularly review the path that the therapy is taking.

The present and too common procedure of deriving a treatment plan from a therapist and seeing a psychiatrist for a pharmacologic prescription or "medication check" is promoted by many managed care services, but as a practice it is hopelessly unsuitable. It has led to improper treatments and to many disasters. I hold that such practices are analogous to letting a midwife make all the decisions over childbirth and leaving the obstetrician to provide the anesthesia.

The therapy should be provided by an expert. One can usually judge a therapist's expertise if, before the therapy begins, he or she is willing to explain the process of the therapy, discuss the benefits and potential problems associated with it, and describe just how long it will likely run. The patient should have a contractual sense of the goals and methods of the therapy from the very beginning.

As with any other treatment, some sense of progress should emerge soon into its course. Any suggestion from the therapist that one must always get worse in order to get better should be viewed suspiciously. In fact, if the patient gets seriously worse (e.g., loses a job, drops out of school, needs to be hospitalized), a second opinion as to the nature of the problem and the prescribed therapy must be sought. Short-term reviews of progress (i.e. feedback) during psychotherapy between the patient and the therapist should be standard, and the justification for either progress or its absence should be grasped.

For many reasons, I recommend that CBT be the preferred form of psychotherapy: it has the best record of success, it works in the most natural way, and interactions between the therapist and patient are direct and coherent. By contrast, what trust I had in conflict psychotherapy has been shaken by the false memory disaster and not restored by the emergence of "traumatologists" and a "traumatic memory" specialty. I would not recommend this form of psychotherapy as an initial treatment for anxiety and depression.

If conflict therapy is tried—and I certainly know competent and broadly experienced therapists to whom I've entrusted patients with severe problems in adjusting to difficult circumstances—then it must stay real. Wild presumptions about unremembered events or mysterious proposals about the way the mind works should provoke a consultation with the referring psychiatrist and a consideration of another therapist. Again, given that psychotherapy is a matter of persuasion, one should be wary of therapists who press patients hard to accept a peculiar idea—such as the certainty of an unremembered traumatic experience. Then one should consider whether the therapy has moved from striving to "influence" to striving to "indoctrinate" and, if so, seek another therapist.

Patients need to be encouraged to retain some sense of responsibility for their actions, even in the course of psychotherapy—the Milgram experiments and the false memory craze demonstrate how difficult this can sometimes be. The opinions of any expert on how the world runs or how it is best construed can dominate any of us if we surrender to them unconditionally. That the recovered memory therapists encouraged such unconditional surrender of vulnerable patients to the culture of suspicion led to tragic consequences.

The best therapists have emphasized that the patient's will and capacity for choice are crucially involved in responding to an expert's opinion. This helps make clear that even with psychotherapy one cannot forever abdicate responsibility for injuries to others—such as publicly denouncing a parent or becoming an invalid and burden to all because of "traumatic memories"—by blaming therapy.

Anyone going into therapy should seek out skillful and dispassionate experts. And then, in this arena of influence, both parties must work in a way that sustains a clear and coherent plan and that rather soon proves itself with steady progress toward its goal.

<hr/>

If psychotherapy is not a way of "curing" but a way of "persuading" people to modify their thoughts and behaviors for the benefit of their mental health, what are the features of someone in good mental health that the psychotherapists seek to achieve through treatment? This interesting question has been asked by patients and therapists alike.

If this question is answered, it makes it easier for therapists to explain their aim and for patients to comprehend when and under what circumstances they can expect to shake hands and say goodbye to the therapist. Most patients don't want to be in therapy forever.

Both therapist and patient might agree that simple symptom relief is unlikely to serve as the only endpoint to treatment. If the patient does not develop some sense of what went wrong in the first place, then symptoms of a similar sort will probably return, perhaps in even more serious and distressing form. Patients must learn something about bringing behavioral responses and emotions under control if the therapeutic enterprise is to affect them in a sustained fashion.

There is little or no argument on this point among experienced psychotherapists. The prime aim of most is to extend Frank's concept of mastery so that it encompasses the idea that with therapy the patients will not only recover from their present symptoms but thereafter be prepared to take responsibility for their mental condition and for managing their problems—and their lives—with a minimum of distress and disruption.

This idea has long been shared by philosophers of human prosperity and aspiration. The renowned bioethicist Leon Kass once noted how this sense of responsibility for one's life and what happens in it is as old as the story of Cain and Abel. Psychotherapists refer to it as gaining an "internal locus of control."

The prime and long-term aim of psychotherapy is to help patients recognize that the only real controls they have over their feelings, their behavior, and ultimately the flourishing of their lives are those they exert on themselves—especially over their assumptions and their responses to changing circumstances and awkward situations. This idea was exemplified by Tim Beck in a CBT text concentrating on treating marital and other relationship problems. The book is entitled provocatively and inspiringly *Love Is Never Enough* (1988).

Distressing events are part of every life. And they impose themselves on us all in many ways—from the simplest kinds of irritations and expressions of bad luck to the most serious kinds of disappointments, deprivations, and traumatic losses. But if you always blame your demoralized states on these events and give what is outside your control—such as accidents or the unkindness of others—dominance over your feelings and your behavior, you will always believe that you're a victim with little chance of contributing to your own well-being. Giving one's self over to an "external locus of control" will inevitably make one vulnerable to emotional defeat.

Successful maturation, whether achieved spontaneously or through various kinds of psychotherapeutic guidance, persuasion, or instruction, recognizes this truth: people to a large extent carry the responsibility for their own psychological balance and satisfactions in life. They must strive to strengthen and confirm that assumption in dealing with the events life brings. The alternative is chaos.

The deficit therapies, such as CBT, that attend directly to how self-control is best attained work toward this goal more directly than do the conflict therapies that come at the issue more indirectly by striving to call up memories of past conflicts and defuse them. The distinguished psychologist and expert in CBT Martin Seligman teaches patients how to attain what he calls "learned optimism." And with this in mind he developed a whole set of therapeutic interactions that help patients, particularly those with pessimistic tendencies, see their own responsibility for fighting demoralization when they hit a snag in life.

Robert Louis Stevenson in his essays and poems regularly champions our responsibility for our own happiness in life. "There is no duty we so much underrate as the duty of being happy," he wrote in his wonderful essay "An Apology for Idlers." Many of the best psychotherapists think the same and exert their influence to help people meet that "duty."

Epilogue

since I described early in this book how my first teachers helped me devise an entry into psychiatry, I want to wrap up my tale by noting how that "path less traveled" shaped the psychiatry I practice and influenced what I came to teach. By doing so, I hope to make clear how our group at Hopkins avoided the destructive misdirections described in this book. We had something more to offer our patients and students— something more comprehensive, coherent, and practical. As I'll explain, our approach immunized us against the chase for "memories" and hidden traumas that stirred the MPD and PTSD clinics and that represented the "convulsive death throes" of the Freudian movement, with its "hermeneutic of suspicion."

For me personally, though, once I had begun to move toward the empirical approach, inductive reasoning, and rational treatments of my first teachers, any attraction I might have had to Freudian thought and practice simply fell away. The patients I saw—initially in the neurological clinics of the Massachusetts General Hospital and then on the services of the Institute of

Psychiatry in London—did not fit with Freudian ideas. Their problems were not that mysterious, and although we psychiatrists in the early 1960s were limited in our therapeutic tools, our patients' difficulties and deficits were best managed by freeing them from confusion rather than by rummaging around trying to bring memories of past conflicts and traumas to their minds.

With this experience I became convinced that Freudian psychoanalysis was more an anomaly than a living tradition with a future. Practical psychiatrists, I believed, would abandon efforts to decode mental disorders as disguised and repressed conflicts and turn to identifying them as psychological impairments and deviations distinct in their origins and open to direct treatment. When my students and I eventually settled at Johns Hopkins, we confronted these issues from a strong position and in a fundamental fashion.

My main efforts were devoted to identifying and describing the differing ways of disrupting mental life. I thought this endeavor crucial because, with the prolonged dominance of Freudian psychoanalysis, psychiatrists had disregarded several alternative explanations for the generation of mental disorders and what they implied. I planned to demonstrate that psychiatric disorders could be gathered into distinct sets according to their derivation. I wanted to emphasize what was already known, identify issues crying out for research, and lay out the more promising directions our group should follow.

In this way I concentrated on building a conceptual structure that sought to make sense of the diverse forms of mental impairment. Let me explain just what that structure entailed.[1]

I proposed that mental disorders fall into four well-defined "families" ("classes" or "metagroups," if you like, or "reference classes," as James Franklin[2] might call them). The disorders encompassed within each family resemble each other in their essential nature. Psychiatrists might still have much to learn about any individual disorder, but if they can identify the family into which the disorder falls, they can sense, from family resemblances, the best directions to follow in searching for its specific cause and a treatment plan most likely to help.

The first family is the class of diseases. The disorders encompassed within this class are those that derive from structural or functional injury to the brain disrupting psychological faculties such as consciousness, memory,

Frame work [handwritten marginal annotation]

230

intellect, perception, and mood. The individual disorders embraced by this family include dementia, delirium, schizophrenia, bipolar disorder, and the like. The aim of research is to reveal the brain changes essential to each of these disorders. At the level of clinical practice, a psychiatrist appreciates that the patient is mentally disturbed because of something he or she "has." Treatments strive to cure or ameliorate it.

The second family is the class of dimensional disorders. It identifies those patients who suffer because of some aspect of their psychological makeup or constitution—weakness of intellect, overly strong emotions, or extremes of introversion or extraversion—that renders them more vulnerable than the average person to life stresses. The patient is seeking help because of who he or she "is." Treatments strive to guide and strengthen such patients in their quest for stability and life direction.

The third family is the class of behavioral disorders. It encompasses conditions such as alcoholism, drug addiction, anorexia nervosa, sexual disorders, and also the hysterical illness-imitating behaviors that I discussed in previous chapters. Here the presenting difficulties derive from what the patient is "doing." Treatments strive to interrupt the behavior and help keep the patient from relapsing into it.

The fourth and final family is that of "life-story" disorders. It encompasses the personal psychological responses to distressing life experiences. The disorders in this family include states of mind such as grief, homesickness, and jealousy as well as the demoralized states emphasized in the last two chapters. Here the clinical problems rest upon what the patient has "encountered" and how he or she is dealing with it. Treatments are directed toward helping them through the distress and overcoming any long-term detrimental psychological attitudes or assumptions derived from it.

This structure of reasoning identified a crucial fact about mental disorders that most psychiatrists with a broad experience already knew. A given symptom—say depression or anxiety—can emerge from any one of these four families, and it is this source of the symptom rather than its manifest character that determines its apt treatment.

A patient could display a depressed mood because he or she has bipolar disorder, because of pessimistic attributes of personality, because of being sickened and discouraged by an alcohol habit, or because of suffering a life-altering disappointment. The patient would look equally depressed, but the psychiatrist planning to prescribe an appropriate treatment must identify the source and so differentiate the nature of the clinical problem. To satisfy that responsibility, a psychiatrist must know the patient well, and this means gaining a full history, including information from relatives, and considering many alternatives in designing a combination of medication and psychological treatment appropriate to the problem at hand.

This approach, which recognizes that similar distressful mental symptoms can have several different sources and that psychiatric disorders fall into distinct natural groups, removes a great deal of mystery from the discipline. It draws upon concepts about human mental life that are well-defined and psychologically coherent.

Our experience at Hopkins has demonstrated that patients appreciate being informed about the family of conditions to which their problem belongs. Again, for them such information dispels much of the mystery surrounding their disorder. They report that knowing that their symptoms derive from, say, some aspect of their temperament or some afflicting illness does much to forge the therapeutic alliance needed for a collaborative effort at overcoming their condition.

This is hardly a new or startling idea. Medical patients gain from learning what type of illness—infectious, metabolic, nutritional, and so forth—explains their physical symptoms, and with that information they can collaborate more purposefully with a treatment plan.

But what's more, our practice of identifying these different sources of mental symptoms helped me grasp quickly—once my attention was drawn to it—what was fundamentally lacking in the MPD and recovered memory clinics (and now among those exaggerating the incidence of PTSD). The champions of these practices failed their patients primarily because they were single-minded. Lacking—or ignoring—alternative ways of explaining their patients' symptoms, they failed to study them thoroughly, were satisfied with surmises, took information out of context, and essentially gussied up the old ideas of Freud to match the contemporary cultural suspicions about childhood and family life.

As my colleagues and I became more familiar with the advantages to practice and research of identifying mental disorders by their essential natures,
and as we witnessed the misdirections of the single-minded, we grew more
insistent in calling for reform of *DSM*. Its classificatory system had served
a purpose when it first appeared in 1980, but unquestionably it also played
a role in supporting the MPD and PTSD misadventures that followed. In
retrospect, such unfortunate outcomes might have been anticipated from
classifications resting primarily on symptoms.

As mentioned in Chapter 9, *DSM* functions as a naturalist's field guide.
It even includes, as an appendix, several "Decision Trees for Differential
Diagnosis" directing the practitioner along observational lines when seeking
the "official" diagnosis for a patient complaining of some common mental
symptoms. These decision trees work like the Twenty Questions game:
animal or mineral? warm-blooded or cold-blooded? feathered or furred?
And so on down the line to a decision.

One such "decision tree" in *DSM-IV* guides the practitioner working
with an anxious patient through the Twenty Questions approach using the
symptoms, their periodicity, their duration, and other such features.[3] In this
way, the psychiatrist is led to distinguish the likes of panic disorder, social
phobia, and generalized anxiety disorder. These psychiatric decision trees
replicate for patients the process by which a wildflower field guide permits
one to use leaf shape, flower color, and the number of blooms to distinguish
among the wild lilies, such as the trout lily, the common fawn lily, the wild
hyacinth, and the wild lily-of-the-valley. Not a useless, but hardly a thorough way of understanding either the fearful or the flowers.

When striving to explain why this approach, which seems at first so
simple and direct, ultimately hinders our discipline, I've used an analogous experience described by a literary scientist. Vladimir Nabokov, in his
captivating memoir *Speak, Memory* (1951), recounts his work as a lepidop-
terist investigating butterflies and moths. Early in his career he also faced
problems derived from the method of classification in use—one that identified butterflies by their color, shape, and flight pattern. He referred to this
system as the "philately-like" or stamp collector's method of study.

He noted that this method appealed to amateur naturalists because it enabled them to put official names to the butterflies they encountered when rambling out of doors. It also put few demands upon the professionals other than memorizing these defining patterns. But, as Nabokov explained, many butterflies look alike in color, shape, and flight and so were by this method erroneously considered identical.

Microscopic study of anatomical structures along with the study of the environmental niches the insects occupy and the climatic and other physical challenges they overcome demonstrated that many look-alikes differ fundamentally—belonging to different species with quite distinct evolutionary backgrounds. This rich understanding eluded the "philatelists." Nonetheless, because of the advantages they found in the simple and popular method, they resisted Nabokov's demands for a more fundamental approach to identification and classification and hindered the advance of the discipline.

I use this analogy when explaining why psychiatrists stick with *DSM-III/ IV*. They like the fact that using its symptomatic definitions guarantees that their diagnoses will survive any challenge. And they (along with other mental health providers) certainly know that differentiating their patients using *DSM* diagnostic criteria demands but a modest effort from them. Even if they realize that *DSM* has them acting like stamp collectors, they often know no better way of assessing their patients.

The truth is that human beings have only a few ways to register, respond to, and report their mental unrest. Not only will those psychiatrists tied to *DSM* symptom profiles in their clinical work fail to distinguish important varieties of mental disorders from one another, but they will continue to confuse the real with counterfeit conditions, as exemplified in their frequent overdiagnosis of PTSD.

The fundamental reason we at Hopkins encourage other psychiatrists (including *DSM* classifiers) to follow our lead and discriminate mental disorders according to the families that provoke them (disease, dimensions, behaviors, life encounters) is that when using this method, psychiatrists must study their patients more thoroughly and get behind their symptomatic appearance. This helps them avoid the misdirections of single-minded explanations and their therapies.

Other ways of mischaracterizing mental disorders will emerge unless the editors of *DSM* learn these lessons of the recent past. *DSM-V*, due to be published in 2012, should (but probably won't) move beyond the stamp collector's method and begin to group mental disorders into natural groups. Our proposal of four groups is a challenge to these officials to produce something of the kind.

Essentially, though, I've told this story because I realize that changing psychiatric thought and practice in these ways will be easier if everyone agrees about just how disastrous to patients and to the psychiatric profession the practice of seeking hidden memories became, and why a field guide manual did not and could not challenge that practice. By drawing attention to the practice I'm not simply recalling the past but identifying a misdirection that continues to this day as evidenced by MPD mutating into PTSD and the latter diagnosis spreading boundlessly in contemporary military and civilian psychiatric populations.

I want all to see how the various therapies built on suspicion, from the earliest forms of Freudian psychoanalysis right up to some contemporary therapies for PTSD, have regularly distracted psychiatrists and kept them from knowing their patients thoroughly—who they are, what they suffer from, and what treatments they need. Only with understanding that begins "where the patient is" can disasters of the sort I've recounted be avoided by psychiatrists in the future.

And as for patients, if they can be helped to comprehend what psychiatrists know and how they know it, they will reject practices built on mysteries and unwarranted suspicions and happily turn to treatment methods with lucid premises and proven benefits. Again, my whole intent in writing this book has been to explain the issues and to hasten the day when coherence reigns in my discipline.

Notes

Chapter 1

1. W. Mayer-Gross; E. Slater; M. Roth, *Clinical Psychiatry*, 3rd ed. (London: Baillière, Tindall & Cassell, 1969), p. 113.

2. Frank W. Putnam, *Diagnosis and Treatment of Multiple Personality Disorder* (New York: Guilford Press, 1989), p. 297.

Chapter 2

1. See Frederick Crews, *Follies of the Wise* (Emeryville, CA: Shoemaker & Hoard, 2006), p. 48.

2. Sir William Osler, "Chauvinism in Medicine," *Montreal Medical Journal* 31 (1902): 684.

Chapter 3

1. M.F. Folstein; S. Folstein; P.R. McHugh, "'Mini-Mental State': A Practical Method for Grading the Cognitive State of Patients for the Clinician," *Journal of Psychiatric Research* 12 (1975): 189–198

2. Richard J. McNally, *Remembering Trauma* (Cambridge, MA: Belknap Press of Harvard University Press, 2003).

Chapter 4

1. Paul R. McHugh, Harold I. Lief, Pamela P. Freyd, and Janet M. Fetkewicz, "From Refusal to Reconciliation: Family Relationships after an Accusation Based on Recovered Memories," *Journal of Nervous and Mental Disease* 192 (August 2004): 525–31.

2. E. F. Loftus and J. E. Pickrell, "The Formation of False Memories," *Psychiatric Annals* 25 (1995): 720–25.

Chapter 6

1. Linda Meyer Williams, "Recall of Childhood Trauma: A Prospective Study of Women's Memories of Child Sexual Abuse," *Journal of Consulting and Clinical Psychology* 62 (1994): 1167–76.

Chapter 7

1. Of some interest is the evolution of the title of the organization that has encouraged MPD and the concept of dissociation in the public. It began as the International Society for the Study of Multiple Personality and Dissociation; then, when the MPD business became problematic, it turned to calling itself the International Society for the Study of Dissociation; and then, when it needed a real justification, it became the International Society for the Study of Trauma and Dissociation. All this name-changing is more public relations and propaganda than progress, given that it is not obvious from the written reports I have read or discussions I have heard that anything has been learned from the huge mistakes perpetrated by MPD and recovered memory therapists. The group has not taken responsibility for the egregious errors practiced by its members and others whom it has taught. It either maintains that the errors were a result of incompetence on the part of some of the therapists, or—when confronted by its own errors—it blames the patient.

2. Sigmund Freud, *Civilization and Its Discontents*, trans. Joan Riviere (London: Hogarth Press, 1930), p. 69.

3. H. R. Trevor-Roper's great essay, "The European Witch-craze of the Sixteenth and Seventeenth Centuries," can be found in *Religion, the*

Reformation, and Social Change (London: Macmillan, 1967).

Chapter 8

1. Nolan D. C. Lewis, *Outlines for Psychiatric Examinations*, 3rd ed. (Albany: New York State Department of Mental Hygiene, 1943), p. 11.

2. Ibid., p. 14.

Chapter 9

1. The *Diagnostic and Statistical Manual of Mental Disorders* (*DSM*) of the American Psychiatric Association (APA) published its first edition, *DSM-I*, in 1952 and its second edition, *DSM-II*, in 1968. Both of these editions are small, almost pamphlet-sized publications that provide diagnostic terms and definitions of psychiatric disorders based on professional assumptions of the nature of these disorders. Beginning with the third edition, *DSM-III*, which appeared in 1980, the manual abjured all efforts to base the diagnostic definitions on anything other than the symptoms and course of the conditions, believing this "a-theoretical" approach improved on the reliability of psychiatric diagnoses. The fourth edition, *DSM-IV*, published in 1994, uses the same approach but adds more diagnostic entities. Both *DSM-III* and *DSM-IV* are large volumes. In this chapter, when I refer to these two volumes jointly as *DSM-III/IV*, I mean to indicate their common approach and the benefits and problems they share because of it.

2. As a wonderfully developed study of how *DSM-III* has, through constructing an overinclusive category, misdirected psychiatric practice and understanding with respect to patients diagnosed with major depression, see Allan V. Horwitz and Jerome C. Wakefield, *The Loss of Sadness: How Psychiatry Transformed Normal Sorrow into Depressive Disorder* (Oxford: Oxford University Press, 2007).

Chapter 10

1. A transcript of the interview can be found in Mikkel Borch-Jacobsen, "Sybil—The Making and Marketing of a Disease: An Interview with Herbert Spiegel," in *Freud Under Analysis: History, Theory, Practice: Essays in Honor of Paul Roazen*, ed. Todd Dufresne (Northvale, NJ: Jason Aronson, 1997), pp. 179–96.

2. Richard Hunter and Ida Macalpine, *Three Hundred Years of Psychiatry,*

1535–1860: A History Presented in Selected English Texts (London: Oxford University Press, 1963), p. 222.

3. Marion L. Starkey, *The Devil in Massachusetts: A Modern Inquiry into the Salem Witch Trials* (New York: Alfred A. Knopf, 1949), pp. 222–23.

4. Henri F. Ellenberger, *The Discovery of the Unconscious: The History and Evolution of Dynamic Psychiatry* (New York: Basic Books, 1970), p. 63.

Chapter 11

1. For an interesting consideration and accessible discussion of the logic of words' meanings and the confusions of purpose they can generate, Martin Gardner's *The Annotated Alice* (New York: World Publishing Company, 1963) is a gem.

2. Otto Fenichel, *The Psychoanalytic Theory of Neurosis*, 50th anniversary ed. (New York: W. W. Norton, 1996), pp. 216–18.

3. Pierre Janet, *The Major Symptoms of Hysteria* (New York: Macmillan, 1907), p. 332.

4. See Mark Pendergrast, *Victims of Memory: Incest Accusations and Shattered Lives*, 2nd ed. (Hinesburg, VT: Upper Access, 1996), pp. 502–4.

5. McHugh et al., "From Refusal to Reconciliation," p. 529. One of the good reasons for seeing the whole phenomenon of recovered memories and multiple personality diagnosis as a craze is that it followed the course of crazes described by Lionel S. Penrose, the British pioneering geneticist and polymath, in a small book, *On the Objective Study of Crowd Behavior* (London: H. K. Lewis, 1952). In it, he identifies, with particular reference to medical practices, how crazes come and go along a similar course, especially when launched with great energy tied either to optimism about cure or anger about harm. Crazes of this sort will work themselves out with a tempo tied to how they are promulgated and how they are confronted. But the sequence of phases is remarkably similar.

    The first phase in the sequence is the latent phase, where the idea is held by a few individuals who are trying to spread awareness of it to the public. They are small in number at first but usually vehement in their convictions, particularly if they derive some energy from other political forces. The latent phase with MPD and recovered memories began with Cornelia Wilbur and her supporters in the early 1970s and can be considered to extend from the time the book and movie *Sybil* drew attention to the claims of child abuse to 1983, when the International Society for the Study of Multiple Personality and Dissociation (ISSMP&D) was founded.

The latent phase of a craze is followed by the explosive phase, where the idea spreads quickly within a community of interested and concerned parties who join together in cultivating the idea, transmitting it through various modes and media into the culture, drawing in more and more support from all kinds of individuals—some directly involved, but many others "fellow travelers" who have social influence and are persuaded by the message. With the MPD and recovered memory craze, the explosive phase ran from about the time of the founding of the ISSMP&D until the mid-1990s. During this phase, many therapists took up the MPD ideas in their practice and some academic psychiatric departments joined in and began to teach these ideas to students. One "fellow traveler" drawn into supporting the craze was the American philosopher Daniel C. Dennett—he with the self-assumed cognomen "bright" (coined by a couple of Californians for people with a naturalist as opposed to supernaturalist worldview).

In the July 12, 2003, edition of the *New York Times*, Dennett wrote: "We brights don't believe in ghosts or elves or the Easter Bunny—or God." But he at least does believe in multiple personality disorder as a product of trauma. In his book *Consciousness Explained* (Boston: Little, Brown, 1991), he identifies MPD and claims to know that "it almost invariably owes its existence to prolonged early child abuse, usually sexual, and of sickening severity" (p. 420). This "bright" ignored the possibility that MPD could be an artifact constructed from social assumptions and contemporary idioms.

The third phase in a typical craze is the saturation phase, in which all the susceptible individuals in the community have been reached such that the market is saturated and the rate of new converts to the craze slackens. With MPD, this phase is difficult to delimit because the severe damage being done by the practitioners precipitated the fourth phase before a social saturation or equilibrium was reached or could be identified.

The fourth phase of a craze is the immunity phase, in which resistance to the idea grows in the community and as a result enthusiasm for it wanes even among those who were initially involved. The MPD craze entered its immunity phase when the practitioners were hit by a combination of strong criticisms from clinicians and scientists such as myself; the formation of the FMSF, which publicized important scientific criticisms; the backlash from many family tragedies produced by the therapists' cruel practices; and eventually severe penalties and sharp rebukes to these practices from the civil and malpractice courts.

From 1992, with the formation of the FMSF, the resistance to recovered memory therapies rapidly increased. By April 1994, the comic strip *Doonesbury* displayed an amusing fictional character, Dr. Dan Asher, described in the strip as "leading guru of the recovered memory movement," who, in explaining the "discoveries," admits, "I had to sue Mom."

The last phase of a craze is its stagnant phase, where the idea fades away except in the minds of a few enthusiasts who may still speak up for the idea and provoke occasional local outbreaks. This is the phase that the MPD and recovered memory craze is in now. On occasion, a case will pop up and the old voices will be heard in the newspapers—but they quickly subside.

6. For a recent review, see Yacov Rofé, "Does Repression Exist? Memory, Pathogenic, Unconscious, and Clinical Evidence," *Review of General Psychology* 12 (March 2008): 63–85.

Chapter 12

1. David A. Alexander and Andrew Wells, "Reactions of Police Officers to Body-Handling after a Major Disaster: A Before-and-After Comparison," *British Journal of Psychiatry* 159 (1991): 547–55.

2. A. C. McFarlane, "The Aetiology of Post-Traumatic Morbidity: Predisposing, Precipitating and Perpetuating Factors," *British Journal of Psychiatry* 154 (1989): 221–28.

3. William E. Copeland, Gordon Keeler, Adrian Angold, and E. Jane Costello, "Traumatic Events and Posttraumatic Stress in Childhood," *Archives of General Psychiatry* 64 (2007): 577–84 (quotation from p. 577).

4. L. Pankratz and J. Lipkin, "The Transient Patient in a Psychiatric Ward: Summering in Oregon," *Journal of Operational Psychiatry* 9 (1978): 42–47.

5. Richard J. McNally, Richard A. Bryant, and Anke Ehlers, "Does Early Psychological Intervention Promote Recovery from Posttraumatic Stress?" *Psychological Science in the Public Interest* 4 (November 2003): 45–79.

6. David Spiegel, "Recognizing Traumatic Dissociation," *American Journal of Psychiatry* 163 (April 2006): 566–68.

7. Institute of Medicine, *Posttraumatic Stress Disorder: Diagnosis and Assessment* (Washington, DC: National Academies Press, 2006), p. 46. See also the editorial by Robert L. Spitzer, Gerald M. Rosen, and Scott O. Lilienfeld, "Revisiting the Institute of Medicine Report on the Validity of Posttraumatic Stress Disorder," *Comprehensive Psychiatry* 49 (2008): 319–20.

Chapter 13

1. Judith L. Herman, in her Guttmacher Award Lecture entitled "Crime and Memory" given at the APA convention in May 1994, described how she wants herself and others to behave after recovering memories of early life trauma and abuse in their patients. She said: "When after [their] careful reflection, our patients do make the decision to speak publicly and to seek justice, we will be called upon to stand with them. I hope we can show as much courage as our patients do. I hope we will accept the honor of bearing witness and stand with them when they declare 'We remember the crimes committed against us. We remember, we are not alone, and we are not afraid to tell the truth.'"

In the same lecture, though, she remarked: "As therapists we are not detectives. We are not fact finders. Our job is to help our patients make meaning out of their experiences."

Somehow the contradictions ("mak[ing] meaning" trumps fact-seeking) did not strike Dr. Herman, but they call to mind an important and classic work in sociology. The German sociologist Max Weber, in his essay "Phenomenology of Sociopolitical Actions: A Methodological Approach to Conflict," distinguishes between an "ethic of responsibility" (*Verantwortungsethik*) and an "ethic of conviction" (*Gesinnungsethik*).

By an "ethic of responsibility," Weber means to identify actions that are undertaken with serious consideration given to their consequences and that demonstrate by strict conformity to professional standards a commitment to accountability. By an "ethic of conviction," he means to identify actions that derive from and are inspired by personally valued ideals. These are to be expressed in the conduct itself and proclaimed in an emblematic way. In the Guttmacher lecture extracts, we can say that Dr. Herman is expressing and encouraging an ethic of conviction and perhaps attending less to matters of professional standards and responsibility.

Doctors and other professional people usually want to reflect both responsibility and convictions in their actions. They trust in professional standards and strive to be sure that the convictions on which they act are professional in the sense of being standards for the task for which they are hired.

More than other doctors, psychiatrists may be attuned and thus vulnerable to cultural assumptions. They may succumb to them when proposing provocations, diagnoses, and treatment plans—even going so far as to ignore the need to confirm the truth.

This power of conviction revealed itself to me every time I asked one of the champions of MPD or PTSD for the evidence behind the diagnosis and receive the response, "You're supporting the aggressors here, you're 'retraumatizing' these poor people by doubting them, you're supporting the Vietnam 'warriors,'" or, as Dr. Herman said, "We're not detectives."

These responses presume either that the truth is so established that further investigation is a bad faith enterprise at striving to sustain a failed position—perhaps a lie—or, and even more professionally unacceptable, that the truth doesn't matter so much as the sincerity on the part of the advocates and the benefits that accrue to the patients—a kind of "antirealist" doctrine tied to cultural politics. If the latter, the presumption would be less a matter of Weberian sociology of conflict and more a penchant of some psychiatrists to present as truth what Harry Frankfurt, the moral philosopher and Princeton professor of philosophy, rightly identifies as (to put it more delicately than he did in a recent book title) baloney.

The therapists who drove MPD forward and the champions of PTSD see their patients in simple ways and work with them from only one point of view—that of victimhood. They do not spend enough time trying to differentiate their patients and are committed to explaining most psychiatric disorders as consequences of traumas, sexual and otherwise.

These shortcomings—and more—tend to occur when professionals let their convictions trump their responsibilities. I would like to say that this failing is unusual, but I can't. In part the carelessness derives from the fact that the *DSM* runs on symptoms alone and thus encourages a checklist approach to diagnosis. In part psychiatrists are to blame because, having grown accustomed to living with convictions built on suspicions, they find it easier to continue following that line than to start gathering facts.

Further exacerbating the problem is that most psychiatrists are pressed by the ubiquitous managed care environment to work quickly and superficially, and the *DSM* offers easy and automatic diagnoses. The time investment with patients that I demand may be too expensive now. Since the APA authorized *DSM*, psychiatrists have only themselves to blame for its part in this sad state of affairs—but that's another book.

2. Michael Shepherd and E. M. Gruenberg, "The Age for Neuroses," *Millbank Memorial Fund Quarterly* 35 (July 1957): 258–65. A full review of this issue, indicating that about 70 percent of patients seeking psychotherapy would recover spontaneously, is found in S. J. Rachman, "The Effects of Psychological Treatment," in *Handbook of Abnormal Psychology*, 2nd ed., ed. H. J. Eysenck (London: Pitman Medical, 1973).

3. This description is from Peter D. Kramer, *Freud: Interpreter of the Modern Mind* (New York: HarperCollins, 2006), p. 102. Elsewhere in this

fascinating book, which strives to be as fair and supportive of Freud as possible, Dr. Kramer makes the following comments: on Freud's treatment of "Dora," quoting Patrick Mahony: "an eminent case of forced associations, forced remembering, and perhaps several forced dreams" (p. 101); on Freud's approach to "Little Hans," where castration anxiety is raised: "a viewpoint whose details are implausible and unnecessary" (p. 119); and on Freud's dream interpretation for the "Wolf Man": "the account is nonsensical" (p. 156).

Epilogue

1. For a full description of the Hopkins approach to psychiatric disorders and their classification, see Paul R. McHugh and Phillip R. Slavney, *The Perspectives of Psychiatry*, 2nd ed. (Baltimore: Johns Hopkins University Press, 1998).

2. For the importance of reference classes in comprehending conditions and rules of evidence, along with their role in the witch craze, see James Franklin, *The Science of Conjecture: Evidence and Probability before Pascal* (Baltimore: Johns Hopkins University Press, 2001).

3. See *Diagnostic and Statistical Manual of Mental Disorders*, 4th ed. (Washington, DC: American Psychiatric Association, 1994), p. 698.

Suggested Reading

Chapter 1

To follow the history of how multiple personality disorder was tied to repressed childhood sexual abuse, begin with Flora Rheta Schreiber, *Sybil* (New York: Warner Books, 1973), and follow up with Frank W. Putnam, *Diagnosis and Treatment of Multiple Personality Disorder* (New York: Guilford Press, 1989), and Carol S. North, Jo-Ellyn M. Ryall, Daniel A. Ricci, and Richard D. Wetzel, *Multiple Personalities, Multiple Disorders: Psychiatric Classification and Media Influence* (New York: Oxford University Press, 1993).

Then turn to the responses: Mark Pendergrast, *Victims of Memory: Incest Accusations and Shattered Lives* (Hinesburg, VT: Upper Access, 1995); Richard J. McNally, *Remembering Trauma* (Cambridge, MA: Belknap Press of Harvard University Press, 2003); Frederick Crews et al., *The Memory Wars: Freud's Legacy in Dispute* (New York: New York Review of Books, 1995).

The best history of MPD from its nineteenth-century origins to the present is Michael G. Kenny, *The Passion of Ansel Bourne: Multiple Personality in American Culture* (Washington, DC: Smithsonian Institution Press, 1986).

Chapter 2

The nature of induction and especially its validity as a method of discerning truth have recently been debated. The best sources dealing with induction as a logical process are Donald Williams, *The Ground of Induction* (Cambridge: Harvard University Press, 1947), and Peter B. Medawar, *Induction and Intuition in Scientific Thought* (Philadelphia: American Philosophical Society, 1969). A book most useful to those interested in the place of induction in the humanistic disciplines is Keith Windschuttle's *The Killing of History: How Literary Critics and Social Theorists Are Murdering Our Past* (New York: Free Press, 1997); see especially pp. 211–21, sections entitled "In Defence of Induction" and "The State of Historical Explanations."

On clinical induction, evidence gathering, and diagnosis, see Allan H. Roper and Robert H. Brown, *Adams and Victor's Principles of Neurology*, 8th ed. (New York: McGraw-Hill Medical Publishing Division, 2005), esp. chap. 1. The original edition of this text was the achievement of Raymond D. Adams and Maurice Victor. Throughout its several editions, including the most recent, it has promulgated and sustained the concepts of reasoning taught by Dr. Adams to medical students and residents at the Massachusetts General Hospital.

For Elvin Semrad's contrasting mode of teaching with presumptions, slogans, and mottoes, see *Semrad: The Heart of a Therapist*, ed. Susan Rako and Harvey Mazer (New York: J. Aronson, 1983).

For the retreat of psychoanalysis into the literary departments of universities and the paucity of its contributions there, see Frederick Crews, *Follies of the Wise* (Emeryville, CA: Shoemaker & Hoard, 2006), esp. chaps. 2–4, where one can find compelling arguments against the Freudian theories delightfully laid forth.

Chapter 4

For an instructive and concise book on Freud and his remarkable influence on our culture, see Peter D. Kramer, *Freud: Interpreter of the Modern Mind* (New York: HarperCollins, 2006).

Informative texts on suggestion and social pressures in memory recovery and MPD are Richard Ofshe and Ethan Watters, *Making Monsters: False Memories, Psychotherapy, and Sexual Hysteria* (New York: Charles Scribner's, 1994), and Elizabeth Loftus and Katherine Ketcham, *The Myth of Repressed Memory: False Memories and Allegations of Sexual Abuse* (New York: St. Martin's Press, 1994).

Those who want to learn why and how Freudian thinking fails as science and as logic can best turn to the classical demolition by Adolf Grünbaum, *The Foundations of Psychoanalysis: A Philosophical Critique* (Berkeley: Unversity of California Press, 1984).

All interested in the acute and chronic effects of traumatic stress should begin with the small treasure by John T. MacCurdy, *War Neuroses* (Cambridge: University Press, 1918), with its fascinating preface by that hero of British wartime psychiatrists who helped Siegfried Sassoon and Robert Graves at Craiglockhart, W. H. R. Rivers.

For how memory works both generally and in relation to trauma, and how it goes wrong with false memories, see, in addition to Richard J. McNally, *Remembering Trauma* (Cambridge, MA: Belknap Press of Harvard University Press, 2003), three books authored or edited by Daniel L. Schacter: *Searching for Memory: The Brain, the Mind and the Past* (New York: Basic Books, 1996), *The Cognitive Neuropsychology of False Memories* (Hove, East Sussex, Eng.: Psychology Press, 1999), and *The Seven Sins of Memory: How the Mind Forgets and Remembers* (Boston: Houghton Mifflin, 2001).

Chapter 5

For studies on the frequency of sexual abuse in childhood and its effects on development and adult life, nothing matches the work of the National Opinion Research Center (NORC) of the University of Chicago. There the most complete national survey on sexual life in the United States was done, ultimately resulting in the publication of two books: one for research scientists and scholars entitled *The Social Organization of Sexuality: Sexual Practices in the United States*, by Edward O. Laumann, John H. Gagnon, Robert T. Michael, and Stuart Michaels (Chicago: University of Chicago Press, 1994), and the other a digested version for the interested public entitled *Sex in America: A Definitive Survey*, by Robert T. Michael, John H. Gagnon, Edward O. Laumann, and Gina Kolata (New York: Little, Brown, 1994).

A fine reference on the history and meaning of MPD and false memory syndrome is Harold Merskey, *The Analysis of Hysteria: Understanding Conversion and Dissociation*, 2nd ed. (London: Gaskell, 1995), and a superb and thoughtful consideration of the whole phenomenon of hysteria is Phillip R. Slavney, *Perspectives on "Hysteria"* (Baltimore: Johns Hopkins University Press, 1990).

What empirical psychological science can bring to the issue of hysteria comes forth in Susan A. Clancy's study on "abductees," *Abducted: How People Come to Believe They Were Kidnapped by Aliens* (Cambridge, MA: Harvard University Press, 2005).

Chapter 6

For definitions of the school of suspicion and the distinctive characteristics of the hermeneutics of suspicion, begin with Paul Ricoeur's book *Freud and Philosophy: An Essay on Interpretation*, trans. Denis Savage (New Haven: Yale University Press, 1970). How suspicion relates broadly to the culture and rests upon hermeneutics is well developed in an article by Erin White, "Between Suspicion and Hope: Paul Ricoeur's Vital Hermeneutic," *Journal of Literature and Theology* 5 (1991): 311–21.

Philip Rieff, *The Triumph of the Therapeutic: Uses of Faith after Freud* (New York: Harper & Row, 1966), classically describes how "psychologizers [as] inheritors of that dualist tradition which pits human nature against social order" (p. 3) affect our culture. The theme of suspicion and what it provides the suspicious was captured well in John Banville's novel *The Untouchable* (New York: Alfred A. Knopf, 1997): "We were latter-day Gnostics, keepers of a secret knowledge, for whom the world of appearances was only a gross manifestation of an infinitely subtler, more real reality known only to the chosen few, but the iron, ineluctable laws of which were everywhere at work. ... for us *everything was itself and at the same time something else"* (p. 45; italics in original).

In describing the contemporary scene and the way a kind of hyper-rationalism has lost touch with reality, with Freud and Marx in particular, I'm inspired by the writings of (and my conversations with) Fred Crews, whose *Follies of the Wise* I've mentioned before. Here I've found delight and inspiration from his wonderful book *Postmodern Pooh* (Evanston, IL: Northwestern University Press, 2006), where he tackles all the confusions in academia and skewers them with wit.

Two superb sources of information about how suspicions carried the day in those awful examples of nursery school and day care prosecutions are Dorothy Rabinowitz, *No Crueler Tyrannies: Accusation, False Witness, and Other Terrors of Our Times* (New York: Free Press, 2003), and the work of two psychologists who brought with them the capacities for thoughtful practice and coherent methods of assessment, Stephen J. Ceci and Maggie Bruck, *Jeopardy in the Courtroom: A Scientific Analysis of Children's Testimony* (Washington, DC: American Psychological Association, 1995).

For the best accounts of particular cases, see Ofshe and Watters, *Making Monsters*, and Loftus and Ketcham, *The Myth of Repressed Memory*, both cited above under the section for Chapter 4. And for a most thorough documentation of cases, see Mark Pendergrast, *Victims of Memory: Incest Accusations and Shattered Lives*, 2nd ed. (Hinesburg, VT: Upper Access, 1997).

Among the best reporting on the Salem witch trials is the recent book by Eve LaPlante, *Salem Witch Judge: The Life and Repentance of Samuel Sewall* (New York: HarperOne, 2007). It depicts the way the emotional presentations of the plaintiffs overwhelmed the defense and the judgment of one good observer who said, "It was awful to see how the afflicted persons were agitated" (p. 136); it also illustrates how resistance and confessions combined to encourage the beliefs of the witch-hunters. The contagion of an idea, a culture of suspicion, and the aloneness of the accused are all vividly drawn.

Chapter 7

For a reasonable but perhaps overly tolerant description of the early developments of the MPD movement and the Mannerist Freudians, see Ian Hacking, *Rewriting the Soul: Multiple Personalities and the Sciences of Memory* (Princeton: Princeton University Press, 1995).

For the growing numbers of therapists and their place in American culture, see Bernie Zilbergeld, *The Shrinking of America: Myths of Psychological Change* (Boston: Little, Brown, 1983), p. 32.

The prompts to the concepts behind the theories of trauma, MPD, child abuse, dissociation as against repression, Janet as against Freud, and reaching into memories are discussed in Henri Ellenberger, *The Discovery of the Unconscious: The History and Evolution of Dynamic Psychiatry* (New York: Basic Books, 1970). Here is where the Mannerists were introduced to Pierre Janet and launched their Freudian heresy. See also Jeffrey Moussaieff Masson, *The Assault on Truth: Freud's Suppression of the Seduction Theory* (New York: Farrar, Straus and Giroux, 1984). And not to be forgotten is that bible of the incompetent therapists: Ellen Bass and Laura Davis, *The Courage to Heal: A Guide for Women Survivors of Child Sexual Abuse* (New York: Harper and Row, 1988).

The mistaken views of laypeople and many mental health practitioners about memory and hypnosis, along with the facts of memory deterioration and retention, are spelled out in detail in E. F. Loftus and G. R. Loftus, "On the Permanence of Stored Information in the Human Brain," *American Psychologist* 35 (1980): 409–20.

The issues of judgment and decision are explored in James Franklin, *The Science of Conjecture: Evidence and Probability before Pascal* (Baltimore: Johns Hopkins University Press, 2001). From his book I have drawn the following comment by Montaigne on witch-hunting and witch trials:

> Methinks one is pardonable in disbelieving a miracle, at least, at all events where one can elude its verification as such, by means not miraculous; and I am of St. Augustine's opinion, that "'tis better to lean towards doubt than assur-

ance, in things hard to prove and dangerous to believe." It is true, indeed, that the proofs and reasons that are founded upon experience and fact, I do not go about to untie, neither have they any end; I often cut them, as Alexander did the Gordian knot. After all 'tis setting a man's conjectures at a very high price, upon them to cause a man to be roasted alive. (p. 57)

Chapter 8

The best examples of how to conduct a psychiatric examination can be found in psychiatric textbooks published prior to *DSM-III* (1980), when checklists of symptoms (sometimes systematic checklists, sometimes random) began to impose themselves on psychiatric assessments. See Lawrence C. Kolb, *Modern Clinical Psychiatry*, 9th ed. (Philadelphia: Saunders, 1977), and Mayer-Gross, Slater, and Roth, *Clinical Psychiatry*, 3rd ed. (London: Baillière, Tindall & Cassell, 1969).

But the source document for the examination is Nolan D. C. Lewis, *Outlines for Psychiatric Examinations*, 3rd ed. (Albany: New York State Department of Mental Hygiene, 1943), which is a revised edition of guidelines first developed by George H. Kirby in *Guides for History Taking and Clinical Examination of Psychiatric Cases* (Utica: State Hospitals Press, 1921). The implications of the "bottom-up" assessment methods described in Lewis's *Outlines for Psychiatric Examinations*, which encourage the recognition of all that a patient brings to a problem—how "every mentally-ill person is a special problem in diagnosis and treatment [because] every patient is a unity, a unique example, suffering from some particular combination of events that has broken or is breaking his adaptations to life" (p. 14)—are crucial to grasp if the MPD, PTSD, and "recovered memory" disdirections are to be corrected.

For evidence that the need for "external informants" is today recognized by the best psychiatric diagnosticians, see Frederick K. Goodwin and Kay Redfield Jamison, *Manic-Depressive Illness: Bipolar Disorders and Recurrent*

Depression, 2nd ed. (New York: Oxford University Press, 2007), where the authors state: "A reading of the relevant literature makes clear that reliable diagnosis of manic-depressive illness requires a longitudinal as well as a cross-sectional view of the patient ... underscoring the need to meet repeatedly with the patient and to seek out other people, particularly family members, who can help in forming an accurate picture of the patient's history, symptoms, and behavior" (p. 89).

The "top-down" diagnostic checklist approach bears much responsibility for contemporary chaos, as Allan Young first recounted in *The Harmony of Illusions: Inventing Post-Traumatic Stress Disorder* (Princeton: Princeton University Press, 1995).

For the important issue of role induction in relationship to psychiatric interventions, the two important papers are R. Hoehn-Saric, J. D. Frank, S. D. Imber, E. H. Nash, A. R. Stone, and C. C. Battle, "Systematic Preparation of Patients for Psychotherapy—Effects on Therapy Behavior and Outcome," *Journal of Psychiatric Research* 2 (1964): 267–81 (where the term "role induction" was first used), and Martin T. Orne and Paul H. Wender, "Anticipatory Socialization for Psychotherapy: Method and Rationale," *American Journal of Psychiatry* 124 (March 1968): 1202–12 (where the importance of the anticipatory socialization process for psychotherapy and how it might work are spelled out).

Chapter 9

For a coherent and fascinating discussion of classification and identification methods in the life sciences, see Ernst Mayr, *This Is Biology: The Science of the Living World* (Cambridge, MA: Belknap Press of Harvard University Press, 1997).

For a full description of how Roger Tory Peterson came to his ideas, how he worked them out with drawings and photography, and just what he accomplished with his field guides to inspire birdwatchers and naturalists in general, see the fascinating recent biography by Elizabeth J. Rosenthal, *Birdwatcher: The Life of Roger Tory Peterson* (Guilford, CT: Lyons Press, 2008).

For all the complicated theories that have affected how we think about the diversity of things that exist, how we might classify them, and what we learn and lose in the various methods we employ, from disjunctive categories to "fuzzy sets," the excellent *Categories and Concepts*, by Edward E. Smith and Douglas L. Medin (Cambridge, MA: Harvard University Press, 1981), can be recommended.

At Hopkins, our doubts about *DSM* and symptom-based diagnosis led to the first empirical challenge of its ways of identifying and distinguishing patients. See J. C. Anthony, M. F. Folstein, A. J. Romanoski et al., "Comparison of the Lay Diagnostic Interview Schedule and a Standardized Psychiatric Diagnosis," *Archives of General Psychiatry* 42 (July 1985): 667–75.

Chapter 10

For matters related to the nature and assumptive world of patients with hysteria, the classic source is Karl Jaspers, *General Psychopathology*, 7th ed., 2 vols., trans. J. Hoenig and Marian W. Hamilton (Baltimore: Johns Hopkins University Press, 1997).

A general review of the generative forces in play in hysteria is Phillip R. Slavney, *Perspectives on "Hysteria"* (Baltimore: Johns Hopkins University Press, 1990); a consideration of all matters related to hysteria—historical, investigative, therapeutic—is Harold Merskey, *The Analysis of Hysteria: Understanding Conversion and Dissociation*, 2nd ed. (London: Gaskell, 1995).

Much contemporary thought on hysteria and the "sick role" derives from the distinguished medical sociologist David Mechanic, developed in several classic papers, including David Mechanic and Edmund H. Volkart, "Stress, Illness Behavior, and the Sick Role," *American Sociological Review* 26 (February 1961): 51–58, and David Mechanic, "The Concept of Illness Behavior," *Journal of Chronic Diseases* 15 (1962): 189–94. Mechanic's concepts were brought further into clinical practice by the efforts of the Australian psychiatrist Issy Pilowsky, in "Abnormal Illness Behaviour," *British Journal of Medical Psychology* 42 (1969): 347–51, and "A General

Classification of Abnormal Illness Behaviours," *British Journal of Medical Psychology* 51 (1978): 131–37.

A most useful paper to consult about the nineteenth- and twentieth-century concepts surrounding hysteria is Mark S. Micale, "On the 'Disappearance' of Hysteria: A Study in the Clinical Deconstruction of a Diagnosis," *Isis* 84 (September 1993): 496–526.

There are many informative references on the Salem witch trials. I've appreciated the book by Marion L. Starkey, *The Devil in Massachusetts: A Modern Inquiry into the Salem Witch Trials* (New York: Alfred A. Knopf, 1949).

A recent and informative close study of the reasoning of one of the judges in the Salem witch trials illuminates just how dramatic testimony tied to contemporary beliefs can overturn judgment and prudence even in the best and the brightest. How convictions can carry responsible people into terrible error is displayed in Eve LaPlante's *Salem Witch Judge: The Life and Repentance of Samuel Sewall* (New York: HarperOne, 2007).

The best source on Mesmer, his methods, and the social context in which he triumphed is Robert Darnton, *Mesmerism and the End of the Enlightenment in France* (Cambridge, MA: Harvard University Press, 1968). Henri F. Ellenberger, *The Discovery of the Unconscious: The History and Evolution of Dynamic Psychiatry* (New York: Basic Books, 1970), also has a fine section devoted to Mesmer.

Many references can be found to Charcot and hysteria in textbooks of psychiatry, but a most helpful source is Georges Guillain, *J.-M. Charcot, 1825–1893: His Life—His Work*, trans. Pearce Bailey (New York: Hoeber, 1959). Not only was Guillain himself a distinguished French neurologist (among other achievements, he identified Guillain-Barré syndrome), but he ultimately held the professorial chair originally created for Charcot at the Faculty of Medicine in Paris. His book contains not only careful descriptions of Charcot's clinic, practices, and thoughts on many matters tied to neurology and psychiatry but also a careful review of the contributions of Joseph Babinski to hysteria and the controversies on the subject that followed Charcot's death.

A vivid, famous, but rather scurrilous description of Charcot at the

Salpêtrière Hospital can be found in the fictionalized autobiography of Axel Munthe, *The Story of San Michele* (New York: E. P. Dutton, 1929).

The emergence of Freudian thought from Charcot, its earliest developments with Josef Breuer, and its implications today are superbly recounted and assessed in Mikkel Borch-Jacobsen, *Remembering Anna O.: A Century of Mystification* (New York: Routledge, 1996).

Chapter 12

Three important books spanning the war-filled twentieth century and vivid in their conceptions of the psychological sequelae to combat are, in chronological order, John T. MacCurdy, *War Neuroses* (Cambridge: University Press, 1918); Lord [C. M. Wilson] Moran, *The Anatomy of Courage*, 2nd ed. (London: Constable, 1966); and Ben Shephard, *A War of Nerves: Soldiers and Psychiatrists 1914–1994* (London: Jonathan Cape, 2000).

A coherent look at the manipulations surrounding the concept of PTSD as the one psychiatric disorder "people like to have" is Derek Summerfield, "The Invention of Post-Traumatic Stress Disorder and the Social Usefulness of a Psychiatric Category," *British Medical Journal* 322 (January 2001): 95–98.

A fine and thorough review of the linkages of concepts and historically proposed mechanisms across all these matters of hysteria, false memories, hypnosis, and PTSD can be found in the book by Michael Trimble, the consultant psychiatrist at the Institute of Neurology, Queens Square, London, entitled *Somatoform Disorders: A Medicolegal Guide* (Cambridge: Cambridge University Press, 2004).

The conceptual foundations of PTSD, the history of "traumatic memory," the emergence of PTSD, and the methods of diagnosis and treatment of the disorder in U.S. veterans hospitals is classically described by Allan Young in *The Harmony of Illusions: Inventing Post-Traumatic Stress Disorder* (Princeton: Princeton University Press, 1995).

The many deceptions tied to Vietnam combat psychological injury and false PTSD claims are revealed in B. G. Burkett and Glenna Whitley, *Stolen*

Valor: How the Vietnam Generation Was Robbed of Its Heroes and Its History (Dallas: Verity Press, 1998).

Again, the book on trauma studies is Richard J. McNally, *Remembering Trauma* (Cambridge, MA: Belknap Press of Harvard University Press, 2003).

For a full assessment of just how the examination of the core concepts of PTSD have collapsed under scrutiny, see Gerald M. Rosen and Scott O. Lilienfeld, "Posttraumatic Stress Disorder: An Empirical Evaluation of Core Assumptions," *Clinical Psychology Review* 28 (June 2008): 837–68.

For a review of the clinical approach to patients exposed to trauma, see Paul R. McHugh and Glenn Treisman, "PTSD: A Problematic Diagnostic Category," *Journal of Anxiety Disorders* 21 (2007): 211–22.

Finally, as a contrast to the way PTSD has been wrestled with, misrepresented, and ultimately made confusing by insisting on its "categorical" nature, consider the thoughtful, coherent, and empirical investigations into grief and bereavement by Colin Murray Parkes, summed up well in *Bereavement: Studies of Grief in Adult Life*, 3rd ed. (New York: Routledge, 1996).

Chapter 13

Hans Eysenck's dramatic challenge in 1960 to psychotherapists (particularly psychoanalytic psychotherapists) that helped launch much of the coherent research into psychotherapy and led to progress in the field is his chapter entitled "The Effects of Psychotherapy" in *Handbook of Abnormal Psychology*, ed. H. J. Eysenck (London: Pitman Medical, 1960). Eysenck's popular books on psychology are also splendid reading on this subject and include *Uses and Abuses of Psychology* (London: Penguin, 1953) and *Fact and Fiction in Psychology* (Baltimore: Penguin, 1965).

The best and most comprehensive description of the nature of psychotherapy is found in Jerome D. Frank and Julia B. Frank, *Persuasion and Healing: A Comparative Study of Psychotherapy*, 3rd ed. (Baltimore: Johns Hopkins University Press, 1991).

Much work on influence and social controls has emerged over time.

Vance Packard was the first and best at describing just how influence can be subtly imposed on us in his classic *The Hidden Persuaders* (New York: D. McKay, 1957).

The experiments of Stanley Milgram are described and discussed in his classic work *Obedience to Authority: An Experimental View* (New York: Harper & Row, 1974). A film of his study entitled *Obedience* is available through the University of Pennsylvania.

A general and useful survey is Robert B. Cialdini, *Influence: The New Psychology of Modern Persuasion* (New York: Morrow, 1984).

Chapter 14

Much of the good sense tied to cognitive behavioral psychotherapy can be found in any of the writings of Aaron T. Beck, who developed the treatment, invested in the research, and tested its protocols. I can recommend a number of books and papers from among a large collection documenting his thought and its foundations. He first described his practice and viewpoint in his classic *Depression: Clinical, Experimental, and Theoretical Aspects* (New York: Harper & Row, 1967). Other sources include *Cognitive Therapy and the Emotional Disorders* (New York: International Universities Press, 1976) and "Cognitive Therapy: A 30-Year Retrospective," *American Psychologist* 46 (April 1991): 368–75. I mentioned his pointedly titled *Love Is Never Enough* (New York: Harper & Row, 1988) in the main text.

For me, the best discussion of and teaching text for CBT, using a case example to demonstrate how it works to challenge pathogenic core beliefs and underlying assumptions, is Judith S. Beck, *Cognitive Therapy: Basics and Beyond* (New York: Guilford Press, 1995).

Martin E. P. Seligman surely is the most creative of psychologists who are directing attention to how assumptions and predilections determine emotional outcomes. He has approached the problem of depressive attitudes from both directions and has added immeasurably to our understanding of that state of mind—first in its form of demoralization and persistence ("learned helplessness," he called it), then followed up on by demonstrations of ways of thinking that lead to recovery and optimism. His classic work on "learned helplessness" is *Helplessness: On Depression, Development, and Death* (San Francisco: W. H. Freeman, 1975). He has described his shift to considering the more positive aspects of mental attitudes in many places, but surely a favorite must be *Learned Optimism: How to Change Your Mind and Your Life* (New York: Alfred A. Knopf, 1990).

Epilogue

To read about what it's like to be on the receiving end of the recovered memory craze as an accused father, see Mark Pendergrast, *Victims of Memory: Incest Accusations and Shattered Lives*, 2nd ed. (Hinesburg, VT: Upper Access, 1997). This book also contains superb descriptions and data about the craze.

Paul R. McHugh, Harold I. Lief, Pamela P. Freyd, and Janet M. Fetkewicz, "From Refusal to Reconciliation: Family Relationships after an Accusation Based on Recovered Memories," *Journal of Nervous and Mental Disease* 192 (August 2004): 525–31, provides comprehensive results of a survey of people drawn into recovered memory treatments.

Index

Other Dana Press Books

www.dana.org/news/danapressbooks

Books for General Readers

Brain and Mind

CEREBRUM 2008: Emerging Ideas in Brain Science
Foreword by Carl Zimmer
The second annual anthology drawn from Cerebrum's highly regarded Web edition, Cerebrum 2008 brings together an international roster of scientists and other scholars to interpret the latest discoveries about the human brain and confront their implications.
Paper •225 pp • ISBN-13: 978-1-932594-33-1 • $14.95

CEREBRUM 2007: Emerging Ideas in Brain Science
Paper • 243 pp • ISBN-13: 978-1-932594-24-9 • $14.95
Visit Cerebrum online at www.dana.org/news/cerebrum.

YOUR BRAIN ON CUBS: Inside the Heads of Players and Fans
Dan Gordon, Editor
Our brains light up with the rush that accompanies a come-from-behind win—and the crush of a disappointing loss. Brain research also offers new insight into how players become experts. Neuroscientists and science writers explore these topics and more in this intriguing look at talent and triumph on the field and our devotion in the stands.
6 illustrations.
Cloth • 150 pp • ISBN-13: 978-1-932594-28-7 • $19.95

THE NEUROSCIENCE OF FAIR PLAY:
Why We (Usually) Follow the Golden Rule

Donald W. Pfaff, Ph.D.

A distinguished neuroscientist presents a rock-solid hypothesis of why humans across time and geography have such similar notions of good and bad, right and wrong.
10 illustrations.

Cloth • 234 pp • ISBN-13: 978-1-932594-27-0 • $20.95

BEST OF THE BRAIN FROM SCIENTIFIC AMERICAN:
Mind, Matter, and Tomorrow's Brain

Floyd E. Bloom, M.D., Editor

Top neuroscientist Floyd E. Bloom has selected the most fascinating brain-related articles from Scientific American and Scientific American Mind since 1999 in this collection.
30 illustrations.

Cloth • 300 pp • ISBN-13: 978-1-932594-22-5 • $25.00

MIND WARS: Brain Research and National Defense

Jonathan D. Moreno, Ph.D.

A leading ethicist examines national security agencies' work on defense applications of brain science, and the ethical issues to consider.

Cloth • 210 pp • ISBN-10: 1-932594-16-7 • $23.95

THE DANA GUIDE TO BRAIN HEALTH:
A Practical Family Reference from Medical Experts (with CD-ROM)

Floyd E. Bloom, M.D., M. Flint Beal, M.D., and David J. Kupfer, M.D., Editors

Foreword by William Safire

A complete, authoritative, family-friendly guide to the brain's development, health, and disorders.
16 full-color pages and more than 200 black-and-white drawings.

Paper (with CD-ROM) • 733 pp • ISBN-10: 1-932594-10-8 • $25.00

THE CREATING BRAIN: The Neuroscience of Genius

Nancy C. Andreasen, M.D., Ph.D.

A noted psychiatrist and best-selling author explores how the brain achieves creative breakthroughs, including questions such as how creative people are different and the difference between genius and intelligence.
33 illustrations/photos.

Cloth • 197 pp • ISBN-10: 1-932594-07-8 • $23.95

THE ETHICAL BRAIN

Michael S. Gazzaniga, Ph.D.

Explores how the lessons of neuroscience help resolve today's ethical dilemmas, ranging from when life begins to free will and criminal responsibility.

Cloth • 201 pp • ISBN-10: 1-932594-01-9 • $25.00

A GOOD START IN LIFE:
Understanding Your Child's Brain and Behavior from Birth to Age 6

Norbert Herschkowitz, M.D., and Elinore Chapman Herschkowitz

The authors show how brain development shapes a child's personality and behavior, discussing appropriate rule-setting, the child's moral sense, temperament, language, playing, aggression, impulse control, and empathy.

13 illustrations.

Cloth • 283 pp • ISBN-10: 0-309-07639-0 • $22.95
Paper (Updated with new material) • 312 pp • ISBN-10: 0-9723830-5-0 • $13.95

BACK FROM THE BRINK:
How Crises Spur Doctors to New Discoveries about the Brain

Edward J. Sylvester

In two academic medical centers, Columbia's New York Presbyterian and Johns Hopkins Medical Institutions, a new breed of doctor, the neurointensivist, saves patients with life-threatening brain injuries.

16 illustrations/photos.

Cloth • 296 pp • ISBN-10: 0-9723830-4-2 • $25.00

THE BARD ON THE BRAIN:
Understanding the Mind Through the Art of Shakespeare and the Science of Brain Imaging

Paul M. Matthews, M.D., and Jeffrey McQuain, Ph.D. • Foreword by Diane Ackerman

Explores the beauty and mystery of the human mind and the workings of the brain, following the path the Bard pointed out in 35 of the most famous speeches from his plays.

100 illustrations.

Cloth • 248 pp • ISBN-10: 0-9723830-2-6 • $35.00

STRIKING BACK AT STROKE: A Doctor-Patient Journal

Cleo Hutton and Louis R. Caplan, M.D.

A personal account, with medical guidance from a leading neurologist, for anyone enduring the changes that a stroke can bring to a life, a family, and a sense of self.

15 illustrations.

Cloth • 240 pp • ISBN-10: 0-9723830-1-8 • $27.00

UNDERSTANDING DEPRESSION:
What We Know and What You Can Do About It

J. Raymond DePaulo, Jr., M.D., and Leslie Alan Horvitz

Foreword by Kay Redfield Jamison, Ph.D.

What depression is, who gets it and why, what happens in the brain, troubles that come with the illness, and the treatments that work.

Cloth • 304 pp • ISBN-10: 0-471-39552-8 • $24.95
Paper • 296 pp • ISBN-10: 0-471-43030-7 • $14.95

KEEP YOUR BRAIN YOUNG:
The Complete Guide to Physical and Emotional Health and Longevity

Guy M. McKhann, M.D., and Marilyn Albert, Ph.D.

Every aspect of aging and the brain: changes in memory, nutrition, mood, sleep, and sex, as well as the later problems in alcohol use, vision, hearing, movement, and balance.

Cloth • 304 pp • ISBN-10: 0-471-40792-5 • $24.95

Paper • 304 pp • ISBN-10: 0-471-43028-5 • $15.95

THE END OF STRESS AS WE KNOW IT

Bruce S. McEwen, Ph.D., with Elizabeth Norton Lasley • Foreword by Robert Sapolsky

How brain and body work under stress and how it is possible to avoid its debilitating effects.

Cloth • 239 pp • ISBN-10: 0-309-07640-4 • $27.95

Paper • 262 pp • ISBN-10: 0-309-09121-7 • $19.95

IN SEARCH OF THE LOST CORD:
Solving the Mystery of Spinal Cord Regeneration

Luba Vikhanski

The story of the scientists and science involved in the international scientific race to find ways to repair the damaged spinal cord and restore movement.

21 photos; 12 illustrations.

Cloth • 269 pp • ISBN-10: 0-309-07437-1 • $27.95

THE SECRET LIFE OF THE BRAIN

Richard Restak, M.D. • Foreword by David Grubin

Companion book to the PBS series of the same name, exploring recent discoveries about the brain from infancy through old age.

Cloth • 201 pp • ISBN-10: 0-309-07435-5 • $35.00

THE LONGEVITY STRATEGY:
How to Live to 100 Using the Brain-Body Connection

David Mahoney and Richard Restak, M.D. • Foreword by William Safire

Advice on the brain and aging well.

Cloth • 250 pp • ISBN-10: 0-471-24867-3 • $22.95

Paper • 272 pp • ISBN-10: 0-471-32794-8 • $14.95

STATES OF MIND: New Discoveries About How Our Brains Make Us Who We Are

Roberta Conlan, Editor

Adapted from the Dana/Smithsonian Associates lecture series by eight of the country's top brain scientists, including the 2000 Nobel laureate in medicine, Eric Kandel.

Cloth • 214 pp • ISBN-10: 0-471-29963-4 • $24.95

Paper • 224 pp • ISBN-10: 0-471-39973-6 • $18.95

The Dana Foundation Series on Neuroethics

DEFINING RIGHT AND WRONG IN BRAIN SCIENCE:
Essential Readings in Neuroethics

Walter Glannon, Ph.D., Editor

The fifth volume in The Dana Foundation Series on Neuroethics, this collection marks the five-year anniversary of the first meeting in the field of neuroethics, providing readers with the seminal writings on the past, present, and future ethical issues facing neuroscience and society.

Cloth • 350 pp • ISBN-10: 978-1-932594-25-6 • $15.95

HARD SCIENCE, HARD CHOICES:
Facts, Ethics, and Policies Guiding Brain Science Today

Sandra J. Ackerman, Editor

Top scholars and scientists discuss new and complex medical and social ethics brought about by advances in neuroscience. Based on an invitational meeting co-sponsored by the Library of Congress, the National Institutes of Health, the Columbia University Center for Bioethics, and the Dana Foundation.

Paper • 152 pp • ISBN-10: 1-932594-02-7 • $12.95

NEUROSCIENCE AND THE LAW: Brain, Mind, and the Scales of Justice

Brent Garland, Editor. With commissioned papers by Michael S. Gazzaniga, Ph.D., and Megan S. Steven; Laurence R. Tancredi, M.D., J.D.; Henry T. Greely, J.D.; and Stephen J. Morse, J.D., Ph.D.

How discoveries in neuroscience influence criminal and civil justice, based on an invitational meeting of 26 top neuroscientists, legal scholars, attorneys, and state and federal judges convened by the Dana Foundation and the American Association for the Advancement of Science.

Paper • 226 pp • ISBN-10: 1-032594-04-3 • $8.95

BEYOND THERAPY: Biotechnology and the Pursuit of Happiness
A Report of the President's Council on Bioethics

Special Foreword by Leon R. Kass, M.D., Chairman

Introduction by William Safire

Can biotechnology satisfy human desires for better children, superior performance, ageless bodies, and happy souls? This report says these possibilities present us with profound ethical challenges and choices. Includes dissenting commentary by scientist members of the Council.

Paper • 376 pp • ISBN-10: 1-932594-05-1 • $10.95

NEUROETHICS: Mapping the Field. Conference Proceedings

Steven J. Marcus, Editor

Proceedings of the landmark 2002 conference organized by Stanford University and the University of California, San Francisco, and sponsored by the Dana Foundation, at which more than 150 neuroscientists, bioethicists, psychiatrists and psychologists, philosophers, and professors of law and public policy debated the ethical implications of neuroscience research findings.
50 illustrations.

Paper • 367 pp • ISBN-10: 0-9723830-0-X • $10.95

Immunology

RESISTANCE: The Human Struggle Against Infection
Norbert Gualde, M.D., translated by Steven Rendall
Traces the histories of epidemics and the emergence or re-emergence of diseases, illustrating how new global strategies and research of the body's own weapons of immunity can work together to fight tomorrow's inevitable infectious outbreaks.
Cloth • 219 pp • ISBN-10: 1-932594-00-0 • $25.00

FATAL SEQUENCE: The Killer Within
Kevin J. Tracey, M.D.
An easily understood account of the spiral of sepsis, a sometimes fatal crisis that most often affects patients fighting off nonfatal illnesses or injury. Tracey puts the scientific and medical story of sepsis in the context of his battle to save a burned baby, a sensitive telling of cutting-edge science.
Cloth • 231 pp • ISBN-10: 1-932594-06-X • $23.95
Paper • 231 pp • ISBN-10: 1-932594-09-4 • $12.95

Arts Education

A WELL-TEMPERED MIND: Using Music to Help Children Listen and Learn
Peter Perret and Janet Fox • Foreword by Maya Angelou
Five musicians enter elementary school classrooms, helping children learn about music and contributing to both higher enthusiasm and improved academic performance. This charming story gives us a taste of things to come in one of the newest areas of brain research: the effect of music on the brain.
12 illustrations.
Cloth • 225 pp • ISBN-10: 1-932594-03-5 • $22.95
Paper • 225 pp • ISBN-10: 1-932594-08-6 • $12.00

Dana Press also offers several free periodicals dealing with arts education, immunology, and brain science. For more information, please visit www.dana.org.